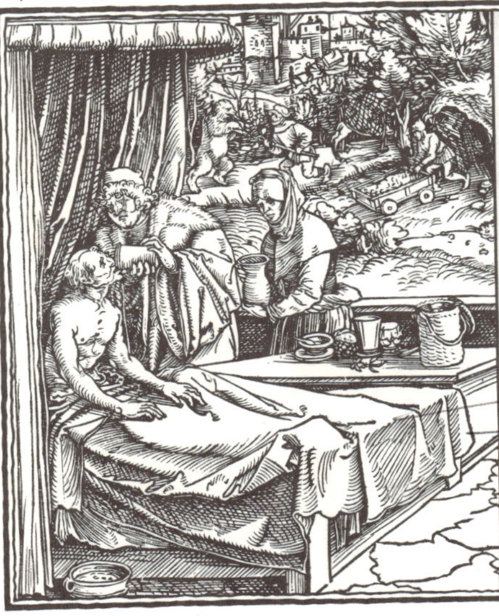

Ex Libris:

Physician ministering
to a patient
(Hans Weiditz).

CANCER IN ATOMIC BOMB SURVIVORS

GANN Monograph on Cancer Research

The "GANN Monograph on Cancer Research" series is promoted by the Japanese Cancer Association. This semiannual series of monographs was initiated in 1966 by the late Dr. Tomizo Yoshida (1903–1973) and is now published jointly by Japan Scientific Societies Press, Tokyo and Plenum Press, New York and London. Each volume consists of collected contributions on current topics in cancer problems and allied research fields. The publication of these monographs owes much to the financial support given by the late Professor Kazushige Higuchi, the Jikei University School of Medicine.

The planning for each volume is done by the Board of Executive Directors of the Japanese Cancer Association, with the final approval of the Board of Directors. It is hoped that the series will serve as an important source of information in the field of cancer research.

Japanese Cancer Association

JAPANESE CANCER ASSOCIATION

GANN Monograph on Cancer Research No.32

CANCER IN ATOMIC BOMB SURVIVORS

Edited by

ITSUZO SHIGEMATSU
Radiation Effects Research Foundation, Hiroshima, Japan

ABRAHAM KAGAN
Radiation Effects Research Foundation, Hiroshima, Japan

JAPAN SCIENTIFIC SOCIETIES PRESS, Tokyo
PLENUM PRESS, New York and London

August 1986

Published jointly by
Japan Scientific Societies Press
2-10 Hongo, 6-chome, Bunkyo-ku, Tokyo 113, Japan
ISBN 4-7622-9490-X
and
Plenum Press
233 Spring Street, New York, NY 10013, USA
ISBN 0-306-42501-7

Distributed in all areas outside Japan and Asia between Pakistan and Korea by Plenum Press, New York and London.

Printed in Japan

PREFACE

Follow-up studies of persons exposed to medical radiation have long shown that radiation induces cancer in man. This, coupled with increasing exposure from other sources including occupational and environmental radiations, has resulted in greater recognition of the importance of research on radiation-induced carcinogenesis and risk assessment with a view to radiation protection.

One of the well-known late effects of radiation is the increased incidence of leukemia that occurred among atomic bomb survivors beginning two or three years after exposure. A remarkable increase of solid tumors including cancers of the thyroid, breast and lung was also observed 10 to 20 years after exposure. Thus, many pathological, clinical and epidemiological studies have been made on radiation carcinogenesis in atomic bomb survivors by investigators at the Atomic Bomb Casualty Commission (ABCC), now known as the Radiation Effects Research Foundation (RERF), as well as by the staff of universities in Hiroshima and Nagasaki. Some of the mechanisms involved in radiation carcinogenesis in man and associated modifying factors, such as age at time of exposure and sex, have been elucidated by these studies. The results obtained are being used by such agencies as the International Commission on Radiation Protection (ICRP) for risk estimations of radiation exposure.

This monograph presents the results realized thus far in these epidemiological and pathological studies. The incidence of radiation-induced cancer among atomic bomb survivors continues to be high 40 years after exposure, and much remains unknown about radiation carcinogenesis. It is hoped that this publication will stimulate the promotion of further studies.

Questions were raised recently on the dosimetry system which has been used as the basis for estimating the risks of carcinogenesis in atomic bomb survivors. As a consequence, a joint reassessment was undertaken some years ago by the U. S. and Japan.

It had been hoped that this radiation dosimetry reassessment, the status of which was reported and discussed at workshops in 1981, 1983 and 1985, would be available for the analyses presented in this monograph. Regrettably, due to the complex nature of the matter a report at the workshop in March 1986 stated that completion of the task was still several months away. Further delay, therefore, in release of this monograph does not appear justified.

It is clear from earlier reports that the estimated radiation dose from neutrons will be sharply reduced and that the estimated gamma dose will increase in Hiroshima, but will decrease slightly in Nagasaki. The shape of the dose-response curve and magnitude of risk coefficients may be altered slightly, but preliminary analyses based on incomplete data suggest that no major change will occur in the determination of the relation of radiation to cancer occurrence.

Many people have contributed to the production of this monograph. In particular, we wish to commend Dr. Hiroo Kato, Dr. Suminori Akiba, and Mr. Geoffrey Day for their invaluable editorial assistance and Mrs. Merry Y. Uemoto for her expert word processing.

May 1986

I. Shigematsu
A. Kagan

CONTENTS

GANN Monograph on Cancer Research 32, 1986

SAMPLING OF ATOMIC BOMB SURVIVORS AND METHOD OF CANCER DETECTION IN HIROSHIMA AND NAGASAKI

Itsuzo SHIGEMATSU and Suminori AKIBA
*Radiation Effects Research Foundation**

The number of acute deaths in both cities which occurred due to the atomic bombings of Hiroshima and Nagasaki in August 1945 until the end of December 1945 is estimated to be between 150,000–200,000 and the number of survivors identified by the supplementary schedule of the 1950 National Census is 284,000. From among these survivors, a fixed population, the Life Span Study (LSS) sample, was established and has been followed by the Atomic Bomb Casualty Commission-the Radiation Effects Research Foundation (ABCC-RERF). In this paper the sampling methods of the fixed population are explained. Also described is the utilization of the tumor and tissue registries in Hiroshima and Nagasaki, the LSS and the Adult Health Study (AHS) for cancer detection among the fixed population.

Atomic bombs (A-bombs) were dropped on Hiroshima and Nagasaki in August 1945. The damage in the two cities was caused by a combination of heat, blast, and fire. The total area demolished by these causes was about 13 km² in Hiroshima and 7 km² in Nagasaki. The energy of the Nagasaki bomb exceeded that of the Hiroshima bomb, but the burned-out areas of Hiroshima were greater because of differences of topography and of the distribution of buildings (Fig. 1).

The number of A-bomb related acute deaths which occurred before the end of December 1945 is estimated to be somewhere between 90,000 and 120,000 out of a population of approximately 330,000 in Hiroshima and between 60,000 and 80,000 out of about 250,000 in Nagasaki (Fig. 1). These acute deaths were attributable to A-bomb radiation, burns, and/or mechanical injuries.

The Atomic Bomb Casualty Commission (ABCC) was established in the two cities by the United States government in 1947 to initiate follow-up studies on the late health effects of A-bomb radiation. ABCC was soon joined in its studies by a branch laboratory of the Japanese National Institute of Health.

In 1975, responsibility for these studies was assumed by the Radiation Effects Research Foundation (RERF), an independent binational institution equally funded by the governments of Japan and the United States.

A nationwide survey of A-bomb survivors was first conducted in 1950, identifying a total of 284,000 survivors throughout the country. A sample of about 110,000 subjects was selected from among these survivors and nonexposed controls who were resident in Hiroshima and Nagasaki at the time of the survey.

As indicated in Table I, mortality in this Life Span Study (LSS) sample has been

* Hijiyama Park 5-2, Minami-ku, Hiroshima 732, Japan (重松逸造, 秋葉澄伯).

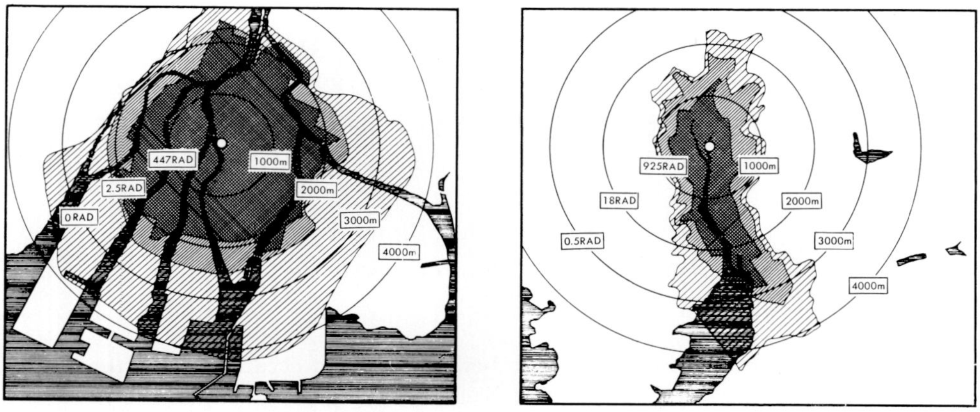

Hiroshima 6 August 1945

Uranium-235 15 kiloton TNT
Estimated population 330,000
Acute deaths during 1945 90,000-120,000

Nagasaki 9 August 1945

Plutonium-239 21 kiloton TNT
Estimated population 250,000
Acute deaths during 1945 60,000-80,000

FIG. 1. A-bomb damage in Hiroshima and Nagasaki. ○, ground zero; ▩, extent of fire; ▨, mean line of structural damage; ▧, limit of structural damage.

under study since 1958, and autopsies (Pathology Study) have also been performed on many of the individuals who have died. Since 1958, detailed biennial medical examinations have been carried out at a participation rate of 75%–85% on an LSS subsample, the Adult Health Study (AHS) sample, comprising about 20,000 members. A separate sample of 2,800 children exposed in utero and their nonexposed controls has been followed for mortality and morbidity.

TABLE I. Major ABCC-RERF Programs

Program	Number of subjects	Year base population obtained	Year study initiated
Survivors			
Life Span	110,000	1950	1958
Pathology	70,000	1950	1962
Adult Health	20,000	1950	1958
In utero	2,800	1945–46	1956
Offspring			
F_1 mortality	77,000	1946–	1960
Biochemical genetics	45,000	1946–	1975
Cytogenetics	33,000	1946–	1967

Program	Type of study	Year study initiated
Other studies		
Immunology	Tumor markers and immune response	1980
Experimental pathology	Cell biology	1979
Cerebrovascular diseases (CVD) (Ni-Hon-San)	Japanese in Hiroshima-Nagasaki, Honolulu, and San Francisco	1969
Cancer	Breast, Lung, Colorectal	1979
Reassessment of A-bomb dosimetry	Japan-US joint study	1981

A large scale genetic study was also conducted based on pregnancy registrations in both Hiroshima and Nagasaki during 1948–53. Furthermore, a sample consisting of 77,000 children whose parents were either exposed or nonexposed was set up in 1960 for mortality follow-up and later for cytogenetic and biochemical genetic studies.

Besides these studies, other programs such as immunological studies and the reassessment of A-bomb dosimetry have been developed (Table I).

Sampling of A-bomb Survivors for Follow-up Study

The earliest, reliable, large sample of A-bomb survivors was defined by the supplementary schedules of the 1950 National Census, totaling about 284,000 survivors, of whom about 159,000 were in Hiroshima and about 125,000 in Nagasaki at the time of the bombs (ATB). Only subjects who were residents of Hiroshima (98,000) and Nagasaki (97,000) in 1950 were used in constructing the Master Sample from which the LSS and AHS subsamples were drawn (*3*). The composition of the Master Sample is shown in Table II. Briefly, the Master Sample consists of two parts; the proper part and the reserve part. The reserve part has the same characteristics as the proper part such as Japanese citizen and known Koseki (family register), but differs in that the Honseki (place of permanent family registration) is outside their immediate environs of Hiroshima or Nagasaki Cities. The proper part was further classified into two parts: "selected" for the LSS sample and "not selected" which was not selected by random sampling in the matching process by exposure distance.

All cases in the Master Sample proper part who were within 2,500 m from ground zero ATB were selected for the LSS sample, with the 28,130 subjects within 2,000 m from ground zero serving as the core of the sample. An equal number of subjects who were between 2,500–9,999 m from ground zero and those not in the cities (NIC) ATB were selected to match the core group by sex and age. However, as the NIC subjects

TABLE II. Proper and Reserve Parts of the Master Sample by Component, Exposure Category, and City

City		Exposure category	Total	Proper part		Reserve part
				Selected	Not selected	
Hiroshima		Total	121,100	74,356	16,341	30,403
	A	0–1,999 m from ground zero	26,174	21,329	—	4,845
	B	2,000–2,499 m	14,543	11,524	—	3,019
	C[a]	2,500–9,999 m	44,478	21,275	14,748	8,455
	D[a]	10,000+m or Not in City	35,905	20,228	1,593	14,084
Nagasaki	Total		42,620	25,037	10,458	7,125
	A	0–1,999 m from ground zero	7,659	6,801	—	858
	B	2,000–2,499 m	5,949	5,144	—	805
	C[a]	2,500–9,999 m	18,152	6,742	8,900	2,510
	D[a]	10,000+m or Not in City	10,860	6,350	1,558	2,952
Total	Total		163,720	99,393	26,799	37,528
	A	0–1,999 m from ground zero	33,833	28,130	—	5,703
	B	2,000–2,499 m	20,492	16,668	—	3,824
	C[a]	2,500–9,999 m	52,630	28,017	23,648	10,965
	D[a]	10,000+m or Not in City	46,765	26,578	3,151	17,036

[a] Matched by age and sex to Group A.

TABLE III. Number of Subjects in the Extended LSS Sample

Exposure		Hiroshima	Nagasaki	Total
Total		82,081	26,679	108,760
Nonexposed (Not in City)		20,170	6,348	26,518
Exposed	0 rad	27,577	4,004	31,581
	1–9	15,933	7,140	23,073
	10–99	13,694	5,473	19,167
	100–199	1,740	1,388	3,128
	200+	1,538	1,369	2,907
	Unknown	1,429	957	2,386

were not available from the 1950 National Census, they were selected from the 1st and 2nd ABCC 10% Sample Censuses in 1950–51 and the 1953 Daytime Census for Hiroshima, the 1950 Listing of Family Heads, the 1950 City Consumer's Registry, and the ABCC 10% Sample Census in 1950 for Nagasaki. Thus, a total of 99,393 subjects constitute the initial LSS sample (Table II). Later, in 1970, all the reserve part of the Master Sample within 2,500 m from ground zero (9,367 persons) were added to the LSS sample in order to enlarge the proximally exposed groups (*6*). Thus, the Extended LSS sample consists of 108,760 subjects as shown in Table III by dose and city.

Another source of information about A-bomb survivors is the A-bomb handbook for which detailed explanation is given elsewhere (*1*). The purpose of issuing the handbook is to identify the A-bomb survivors based on the Atomic Bomb Survivors Medical Treatment Law which was enacted in 1957 for administrative purposes. Information on A-bomb radiation exposure status for the A-bomb handbook is based on the report made by the subject at the time of handbook issue, *i.e.*, 1957 or later. Initially, medical care was limited by the law to the proximally exposed. Later, many persons who entered the cities immediately after the bombing, the so-called early entrants, were also included as A-bomb handbook holders. Thus, the total number of A-bomb handbook holders was about 370,000 as of March 1984 (*1*). It is believed that the exposure information from the A-bomb handbook is less accurate and not as complete as that ascertained for the ABCC-RERF sample. Also, estimation by the most reliable method of exposure dose from A-bomb radiation is virtually limited to survivors belonging to the RERF sample. Thus, the results of surveys referred to in this monograph are limited to those conducted on the ABCC-RERF samples unless otherwise specified.

Method of Cancer Detection

1. Tumor and tissue registry

A) Tumor registry

Tumor Registries were established in 1957 for Hiroshima and in 1958 for Nagasaki under the auspices of the respective City Medical Associations and with the technical support of ABCC (*5*). The specific purpose was to develop and maintain a source of information on tumors diagnosed in these two communities. They have been, and continue to be, effective mechanisms for the collection and storage of cancer case information, and the data recorded have been invaluable in the assessment of the role of ionizing radiation in the etiology of certain specific cancers, particularly nonfatal cancer.

B) Tissue registry

The Tissue Registries are designed to collect and examine surgical tumor tissue from both Hiroshima and Nagasaki subjects. Tumors are classified and the tissues are stored. This procedure permits reexamination of tissues by investigators for specific research projects. The Tissue Registry was established in Hiroshima in 1973 under the auspices of the Hiroshima Prefectural Medical Association (thus the Tissue Registry covers tumor tissue removed during surgery conducted in Hiroshima prefecture including Hiroshima City). A similar Tissue Registry was initiated by the Nagasaki City Medical Association in September 1974.

The information for tumor cases registered in the Tumor and/or Tissue Registry who are LSS members becomes available by checking the names in the registry against the RERF Master File once a year.

The completeness of registration appears to be high, judging from the low proportion of cases which were registered only upon death certificate information (9% in Hiroshima and 7% in Nagasaki). However, overregistration may occur because of the inclusion of doubtful diagnoses, and occult cancer. In order to reduce the false negative rate in screening cases for the cancer registry, a diagnosis described as doubtful by the attending physician is so registered, unless it is corrected or confirmed by a later report. As mentioned earlier, the autopsy rate is high in Hiroshima and Nagasaki, particularly in the RERF sample, so therefore the number of occult cancer (recognized only at autopsy) is also high. The consequence of such overregistration will be described later in this monograph. The Tumor Registry data are limited to sample members who lived in Hiroshima and Nagasaki cities or adjacent areas at the time of diagnosis, whereas the

TABLE IV. Accuracy of Cause of Death—Autopsy Cases among the LSS Sample, 1961–75

Cause of death	Death certificate	Autopsy report	Agreement	Confirmation rate (%)	Detection rate (%)
Tuberculosis	176	226	110	62.5	48.7
Malignant neoplasms of:					
Buccal cavity and pharynx	19	17	13	68.4	76.5
Esophagus	50	53	36	72.0	67.9
Stomach	444	495	374	84.2	75.6
Large intestine	43	54	28	65.1	51.9
Rectum	45	46	32	71.1	69.6
Liver, gallbladder and bile ducts	42	169	26	61.9	15.4
Pancreas	56	81	36	64.3	44.4
Trachea, bronchus, lung	192	172	117	60.9	68.0
Breast	40	49	38	95.0	77.6
Uterus	70	83	57	81.4	68.7
Prostate	13	24	5	38.5	20.8
Urinary organs	38	60	30	78.9	50.0
Malignant lymphoma	40	56	31	77.5	55.4
Leukemia	42	40	36	85.7	90.0
Benign neoplasms and neoplasms of unspecified nature	65	21	3	4.6	14.3
Diseases of blood and blood-forming organs	30	14	12	40.0	85.7
Ischemic heart disease	265	199	67	25.3	33.7
Gastric, duodenal, and peptic ulcer	58	61	24	41.4	39.3
Cirrhosis of liver	153	149	80	52.3	53.7
Nephritis and nephrosis	62	29	11	17.7	37.9

mortality data cover subjects from all Japan. Since migration rates do not differ by radiation dose according to recent analyses of the AHS (*8*), this difference should not cause a serious problem in analysis of radiation induced cancer. However, a more detailed study of this problem of migration will be undertaken in the future.

2. The Life Span Study (LSS): a mortality survey

In Japan, all vital demographic events such as births, deaths, and marriages are registered at the legal address of the family (Honseki). This family registration system (Koseki) has been operating for more than 100 years. Therefore, it is possible to ascertain accurately the survival status of a person by checking the family register through the Honseki regardless of actual residence. Nearly all deaths in the LSS sample have been verified through the Koseki check and the cause of death is obtained from the vital statistics death schedules kept at the Health Center which covers the location at death. As the death certificate is used to prepare the death schedules, the accuracy of the cause classification must be checked against the autopsy report whenever possible. Table IV shows, in terms of confirmation and detection rates, the accuracy of the cause of death classification on death certificates as revealed by autopsy findings for those individuals who were autopsied (*9*). Confirmation rates differ according to the cause of death; the rate is high for cancer such as leukemia, lung, and stomach, being 70%–80%, but the accuracy is poor for cancer such as pancreas and liver where the confirmation rate is less than 50%. In studying cancer of sites having low accuracy, it is possible to restrict the study to only those histologically confirmed either through autopsy or surgical pathology.

The underlying cause of death is classified according to the International Classification of Diseases (ICD). The cause of death was coded by the 7th (1950–67), 8th (1968–78), and 9th (1979 or later) ICD revisions.

3. The Adult Health Study (AHS): a clinical survey

Regular biennial clinical examinations of the AHS sample which began in 1958 are now in the 14th examination cycle (1984). Sample selection and characteristics of the AHS are described elsewhere (*2, 4*). The original AHS population of almost 20,000 included two exposed and two control groups of approximately equal numbers as given in Table V: 1) a group within 2,000 m from ground zero, who reported acute radiation symptoms; 2) another group within 2,000 m, without acute radiation symptoms; 3) a control group between 3,000–3,499 m in Hiroshima and 3,000–3,999 m in Nagasaki; and 4) another control group not in the city ATB. Groups 2, 3, and 4 were matched to Group 1 by age and sex. The examination schedule was set so that in any one month a more or less representative cross section of the entire population would visit the clinic. Over time,

TABLE V. The AHS Sample by Sex, City, and Exposure Group

Exposure group	Hiroshima		Nagasaki		Both cities		Total
	Male	Female	Male	Female	Male	Female	
1. Within 2,000 m with symptoms	1,312	2,116	678	887	1,990	3,003	4,993
2. Within 2,000 m without symptoms	1,313	2,114	677	883	1,990	2,997	4,987
3. 3,000–3,499 m in Hiroshima 3,000–3,999 m in Nagasaki	1,312	2,119	674	885	1,986	3,004	4,990
4. Not in city ATB	1,313	2,120	676	883	1,989	3,003	4,992
Total	5,250	8,469	2,705	3,538	7,955	12,007	19,962

attrition (death, moved from city, and refusal) has reduced the population examined in 1984 to about 50% of the original sample.

The medical examination in the clinic is a standard one, consisting of a system review, physical findings, and up to six diagnoses according to ICD nomenclature, all coded. Other basic clinical data at the time of the examination are systolic and diastolic blood pressure, height and weight, and electrocardiogram and chest film diagnoses, all coded. Ultrasonography of the abdomen, begun in Hiroshima in 1982, is performed regularly on about 50% of the AHS, while of these, 75% also have a thyroid examination, and about 60% (females) a breast examination.

In addition to routine laboratory tests, specific biochemical and immunological assay for cancer screening was recorded. Included among these procedures are serum pepsinogen and anti parietal antibody for stomach cancer and α-fetoprotein and HB-s antigen for liver cancer.

The clinical diagnoses available for the AHS are difficult to characterize, especially if they are not based on laboratory findings. Most investigators have used the coded diagnoses for initial ascertainment only, reexamining the patient or reviewing the medical records to make final selections in relation to study criteria. There is little information on the frequency with which diagnoses are missed. The ascertainment varies also in relation to the special interests and experience of the examiners, the existence of particular substudies, and other factors.

On Limitations of Data

Although these epidemiological studies included control groups for comparative purposes, it was not possible to set up an ideal population sample (7). For example, the number of survivors exposed near ground zero is limited, and cannot be augmented. The selection of a proper control group presents another problem. Essentially, any control group should resemble the experimental group in every respect except the factors being tested (radiation exposure in this case). Because everyone in the area was exposed to some degree and subject to blast effects and burns, a sample was taken of the population residing in the city at the time of the survey who were not in the cities ATB. The NIC group was subdivided into early and late entrants into the cities since they might have represented different kinds of populations. Actually, the NIC group appears to differ from the A-bomb survivors in other respects such as socioeconomic status. Therefore, in many instances, the NIC group has been abandoned as a control in favor of survivors with very low exposure doses, for example, 0, or 0–9 rad.

The studies involving the major samples are based on the A-bomb survivors who were still alive at the initial survey about five years after the bombs. Therefore, the samples exclude the more severely injured, and offer the possibility of measuring the delayed effects of exposure, from light to moderately heavy radiation doses.

Sample size poses a problem. When the data are classified by city, sex, age, radiation exposure, and cause of illness or cause of death, the frequency of events dwindles very rapidly. This introduces variability into the data, and creates difficulties in their interpretation. Inferences can be made only after the performance of statistical tests of significance to give some assurance that the differences observed are not due to chance alone.

REFERENCES

1. A-bomb Casualty Relief Department, Public Health Bureau, Hiroshima City. "Gembaku Hibakusha Taisaku Jigyo Gaiyo, Showa 59 Nen-ban (General Description of Projects to Help A-bomb Survivors, Annual Report 1984)."
2. Beebe, G.W., Fujisawa, H., and Yamasaki, M. Adult Health Study. Reference papers. A. Selection of the sample. B. Characteristics of the sample. ABCC Tech. Rep. 10-60 (1960).
3. Beebe, G. W. and Usagawa, M. The major ABCC samples. ABCC Tech. Rep. 12-68 (1968).
4. Hollingsworth, J. W. and Beebe, G. W. Adult Health Study, provisional research plan. ABCC Tech. Rep. 9-60 (1960).
5. Ishida, M., Zeldis, L. J., and Jablon, S. Tumor registry study in Hiroshima and Nagasaki. ABCC Tech. Rep. 2-61 (1961).
6. Kato, H. and Schull, W. Life Span Study Report 9. Part 1. Cancer mortality among atomic bomb survivors, 1950–78. RERF Tech. Rep. 12-80 (1980).
7. Moriyama, I. M. Capsule summary of results of radiation studies on Hiroshima and Nagasaki atomic bomb survivors, 1945–75. RERF Tech. Rep. 5-77 (1977).
8. Sawada, H., Kodama, K., Shimizu, Y., and Kato, H. RERF Adult Health Study, Report 6. Result of the six examination cycles, 1968–80, Hiroshima and Nagasaki. RERF Tech. Rep. 3-86 (1986).
9. Yamamoto, T., Moriyama, I. M., Asano, M. and Guralnick, L. RERF Pathology Studies, Report 4. Autopsy program and the Life Span Study, Hiroshima and Nagasaki, January 1961–December 1975. RERF Tech. Rep. 18-78 (1978).

GANN Monograph on Cancer Research 32, 1986

ATOMIC BOMB DOSIMETRY FOR EPIDEMIOLOGICAL STUDIES OF SURVIVORS IN HIROSHIMA AND NAGASAKI

Takashi MARUYAMA*
Division of Physics, National Institute of Radiological Sciences

Better atomic bomb (A-bomb) radiation dose estimates with a higher accuracy are required for the epidemiological studies in Hiroshima and Nagasaki. Several scientists have tried to evaluate the free-in-air gamma ray and neutron dose and some weighting factors such as house shielding and body shielding. Since 1965, the tentative 1965 dose (T65D) has been widely used as the basic data for the dose determination of A-bomb survivors in epidemiological studies.

In 1976, however, the reevaluation of the T65D dose was proposed by an American scientist who calculated the A-bomb doses on the basis of declassified data on the radiation spectra of the A-bomb. The development of computer technology made it possible to perform complicated dose-calculations for the Hiroshima and Nagasaki bombs.

This paper describes the history of A-bomb dosimetry, reviews some issues in the determination of T65D, and discusses the necessity of reassessment of A-bomb dose and the expected values for survivors.

By 1955 the Atomic Bomb Casualty Commission (ABCC) had accumulated a large body of medical information on the survivors in Hiroshima and Nagasaki. Most survivors were exposed to the atomic bombs (A-bombs) inside Japanese houses. According to ABCC investigations, Japanese houses were highly uniform in construction such as slope, thickness, and composition of the roofs, thickness and composition of the interior and exterior walls, and type and arrangement of framing. To determine the shielding factors typical Japanese houses were built at the Nevada Test Site and used during dosimetry studies in the Ichiban Project (*3*).

The early dose estimates for each survivor were determined on the basis of the tentative 1957 dose (T57D), the so-called York curves, which made the evaluations using results of A-bomb experiments at the Nevada Test Site (*28*). Since there were large errors in the dose determination because of uncertainties in the yield estimates of the bombs, the location of the explosion points, and various parameters in evaluating shielding, dose estimates with a higher degree of accuracy were desired. To revise the T57D, ABCC, in 1957, asked the Oak Ridge National Laboratory (ORNL) and the National Institute of Radiological Sciences (NIRS) for reevaluation of A-bomb doses. In 1965, ORNL and NIRS determined free-in-air doses for gamma rays and neutrons in Hiroshima and Nagasaki which were used to construct the tentative 1965 dose (T65D) (*24*). The current individual doses of A-bomb survivors in the ABCC/Radiation Effects

* Anakawa-cho 4-9-1, Chiba 260, Japan (丸山隆司).

Research Foundation (RERF) Life Span Study (LSS) sample have been evaluated on the basis of the T65D.

In 1976, Preeg of the Los Alamos National Laboratory (LANL) calculated free-in-air gamma ray and neutron doses, using the neutron and gamma ray output spectra of both the Hiroshima and Nagasaki bombs which were declassified by the US Energy Research and Development Administration and were published as a letter (*36*). Although the results of the dose calculations were not valid, they encouraged scientists to reevaluate the A-bomb doses in Hiroshima and Nagasaki using the declassified output spectra. In 1980, Kerr (*17*, *18*) of ORNL, and Loewe and Mendelsohn (*20*) of Lawrence Livermore National Laboratory (LLNL) calculated free-in-air gamma ray and neutron doses, using the output spectra proposed by Preeg. The ORNL and the LLNL reevaluations of the A-bombs in Hiroshima and Nagasaki were discussed at the Late Effects Workshop on Dosimetry of the Atomic Bomb Survivors (*30*) in 1981. Furthermore, a symposium entitled Reevaluations of Dosimetric Factors, Hiroshima and Nagasaki (*34*), was held under the auspices of the US Department of Energy in 1981 to evaluate past, present, and projected work on the A-bomb dosimetry. At these meetings it was impossible to determine which dose estimate is valid, the T65 dose or the revised dose by ORNL and LLNL. After these meetings, the US committee (Chairman: Dr. Seitz, Rockfeller University) and the Japanese committee (Chairman: Dr. Tajima, Rikkyo University) on reevaluation of the A-bomb doses were almost simultaneously established to decide an agreed best estimate of dose to survivors.

The first US-Japan Joint Workshop for Reassessment of Atomic Bomb Radiation Dosimetry in Hiroshima and Nagasaki was held in Nagasaki in February of 1983. At this workshop, new data on the gamma ray and neutron output spectra for the Hiroshima bomb evaluated with two-dimensional calculations were presented by Whalen (*37*). Kerr *et al.* (*19*) revised the gamma ray and neutron doses in Hiroshima which were previously published, with a dose recalculation on the basis of the new spectra calculated by Whalen. In November of 1983, the second US-Japan Joint Workshop was held in Hiroshima. At the second workshop a dosimetry system for A-bomb survivors including house shielding factors and organ dosimetric procedures was mainly discussed (*27*).

The Tentative 1965 Dose (T65D) Estimates

1. Characteristics of the A-bombs

The Nagasaki bomb was an implosion-type weapon that used thick charges of high explosive to compress a subcritical mass of ^{239}Pu into a critical mass at the time of explosion (Fig. 1). The implosion-type bomb was fired at Alamogordo in July 1945, at the Bikini Able test in 1946, and in several other tests at the Nevada Test Site. The Hiroshima bomb was a gun-assembly weapon that used a small propellant charge to shoot one piece of ^{235}U as a bullet against another piece to create a critical mass (Fig. 1). Since this type of bomb had never been fired at any other time, the dose estimates for Hiroshima were much more approximate as compared with those for Nagasaki. The mass and atomic number of materials surrounding the fissionable core are essential factors for the evaluation of radiation yield and quality. In the Nagasaki bomb, the surrounding materials contained high explosive of which hydrogen and nitrogen slowed down and absorbed most of the neutrons and consequently produced an intense source of high energy gamma rays. In the Hiroshima bomb, the iron and heavier metals used in parts

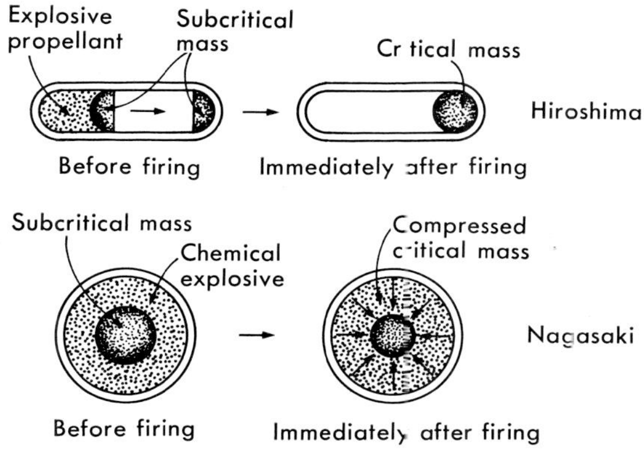

FIG. 1. Schematic illustration of construction of the Hiroshima and Nagasaki atomic bombs.

of the nose and tail of the bomb slowed down many fast neutrons and absorbed gamma rays, so that the neutron doses at corresponding distances from ground zero were thought to be very large as compared with those in Nagasaki. The radiation dose on the ground decreased rapidly with increasing distance from the burst point of the bomb due to geometrical and atmospheric attenuation.

2. *Exponential function for dose estimations*

According to the results of early A-bomb tests (*6*), gamma ray and neutron doses were given as a function of slant distance from the point of detonation at various distances above the air/ground interface by the following equation (Fig. 2):

$$D(R) = \frac{G_0 \exp(-R/L)}{R^2} \tag{1}$$

where $D(R)$ is free-in-air dose in rad at a slant distance R, L is the relaxation length in meters (m) for the type of radiations under consideration at a given air density, and G_0 is the intensity in rad$\cdot$m^2 and is dependent on the particular type of A-bomb, yield, and type of radiation. During the early A-bomb tests, film badges and tetrachloroethylene chemical dosimeters were used to measure gamma ray doses, and neutron fluence distributions were determined with threshold detectors (*2*). It appeared likely that it would be difficult to determine precise radiation doses with these primitive detectors. Figure 3 shows the York curves, which were used for the dose determinations of

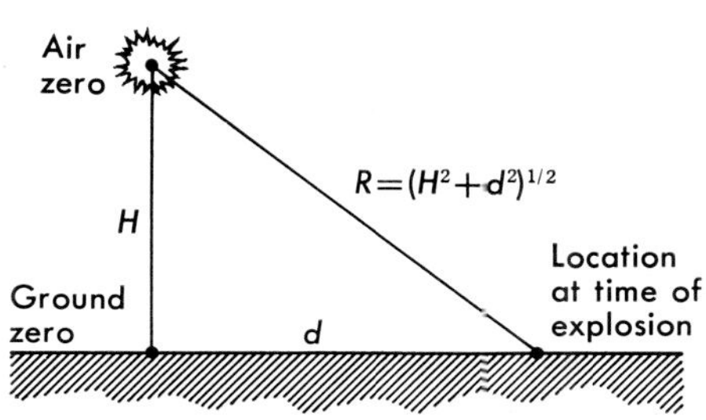

FIG. 2. Slant distance.

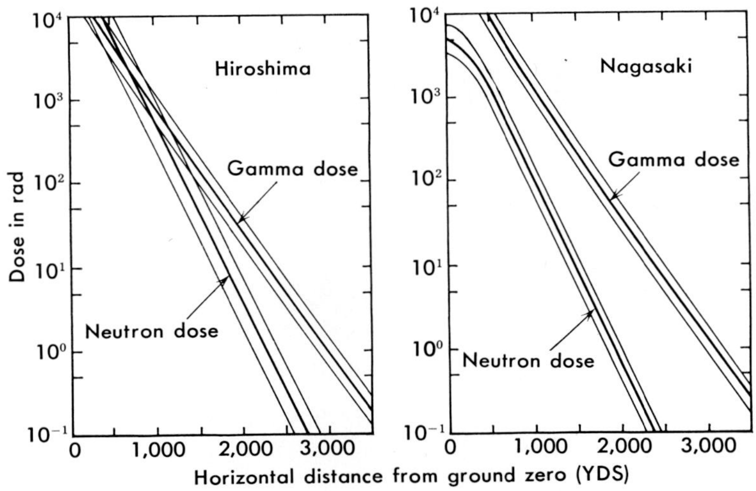

FIG. 3. The York curves for the Hiroshima and Nagasaki bombs.

A-bomb survivors in Hiroshima and Nagasaki up to 1965. The methodology for the determinations of these curves is still unknown.

3. *Operation BREN*

To measure the gamma ray and neutron doses with sensitive laboratory-type instrumentation, the Bare Reactor Experiment, Nevada (BREN) was developed as a part of the Ichiban Project. The main objectives of Operation BREN were 1) to measure gamma ray and neutron doses in Japanese houses, 2) to determine the energy and angular distribution of gamma rays and neutrons, and 3) to measure energy and dose as functions of distance and height.

The Health Physics Research Reactor (HPRR) was designed to simulate the radiation field from an A-bomb. The HPRR was mounted on a 460 m-high tower constructed at the Nevada Test Site, and a ^{60}Co source of a nominal 1200 Ci (1 Ci=a 3.7×10^{10} Bq in SI unit) was substituted for the reactor to compensate gamma rays from fission products markedly attenuated in the reactor. As a part of the Ichiban Project, the LANL constructed a critical assembly designed to have nuclear characteristics similar to those of the Hiroshima bomb. Spectrum and dose measurements of neutrons from the critical assembly were carried out in the laboratory. The gamma ray dosimeter used during Operation BREN was the Phil, which is based on a miniature Geiger counter appropriately encapsulated so that its response per unit dose as a function of photon energy is uniform from an energy less than 100 keV to 10 MeV. The encapsulating shield included ^{6}Li to protect the detector from thermal neutrons to which it has a significant response (*35*). The neutron dosimeter used during Operation BREN was a Hurst proportional counter in conjunction with the appropriate electronics to provide a measure of approximate tissue kerma in air (*14*).

4. *ORNL-Auxier*

Since 1956, Auxier and his co-workers (Health Physics Division, ORNL) have conducted studies in conjunction with ABCC, aimed at determining the radiation dose

TABLE I. Dosimetric Parameters Used for the ORNL Dose Determinations (*3*)

Item	Hiroshima		Nagasaki	
	ORNL (1965)	York (1957)	ORNL (1965)	York (1957)
Energy yield, ktons of TNT equivalent	12.5	18.5	22	23
Height of burst (m)	570	550	500	519
Relaxation length (m)				
Neutrons	198	218	198	218
Gamma rays	250	346	350	346
Extrapolated G_0 at burst point ($m^2 \times rad$)				
Neutrons	8.70×10^{10}	8.64×10^{10}	1.30×10^{10}	1.25×10^{10}
Gamma rays	3.45×10^{10}	2.16×10^{10}	2.75×10^{10}	2.68×10^{10}

York's and Wilson's values of G_0 have been converted to rad·cm² by multiplying by $(0.9144\ m/yd)^2 \times (0.93\ rad/R)$.

Relaxation length is corrected to 1.133 g/*l*., the surface air density in both cities at the time of the bombings.

Wilson gives only neutron fluxes. Values of G_0 for dose have been calculated from his fast fluxes assuming one-fast fission neutron per square centimeter delivers 1.14×10^{-9} rad.

Neutrons above 3 MeV and slow neutrons add only a few percent to the dose.

for survivors in Hiroshima and Nagasaki. They evaluated free-in-air doses of gamma rays and neutrons as a function of distances from ground zero, based on the results of Operation BREN and Ichiban experiments.

In Nagasaki, using the best gamma ray dose estimates from early A-bomb tests and computing a least squares solution, the values of G_0 and L given in Eq. (1) were determined. These values are given in Table I.

In Hiroshima, since no similar bomb had been test fired, the factors of G_0 and L were determined using the results of Operation BREN and the critical assembly experiment. Auxier (*3*) assumed that for gamma rays the relaxation length for neutrons was the same as in Nagasaki, but for gamma rays the relaxation length was much less in Hiroshima than in Nagasaki because of the difference in the construction of the bombs. At that time, they assumed that the energy yield of the Hiroshima bomb was 12.5 ktons of trinitrotoluen (TNT) equivalent and 22 ktons for the Nagasaki bomb. The results of the critical assembly experiment showed that total neutrons per fission was 0.76 and neutron dose per fission was 7.71×10^{-17} rad fission^{-1} at 9.46 m. They calculated the factor of G_0 for Hiroshima neutrons as 1.25×10^{10} rad m^{-2} at 1 m (12.5 ktons $\times 1.45 \times 10^{23}$ fission kton$^{-1} \times 7.71 \times 10^{-17}$ rad fission$^{-1} \times 9.46^2$ m^2). The buildup factor for neutrons was derived from the data measured in Operation BREN and was equal to 6.96. Table I gives the resultant values of these factors.

5. *NIRS and Kyoto University*

In 1961, Hashizume *et al.* (*13*) of NIRS started a project to evaluate free-in-air doses of gamma rays and neutrons in Hiroshima and Nagasaki at the request of ABCC. The NIRS group evaluated the gamma ray doses by thermoluminescent methods, using bricks and ornamental tiles from buildings which were still standing in Hiroshima and Nagasaki. In addition, they estimated the neutron doses from the activation of cobalt in iron reinforcing bars embedded at a depth of about 8 cm from the surface of ferroconcrete buildings in both cities.

TABLE II. Specific Activities of ^{60}Co in Iron Bars and Resultant Neutron Dose (NIRS)

City	Coordinates of samples	Distance from ground zero (m)	Incident angle (°)	Activity[a] cpm/mg Co	Neutron dose (rad)
Hiroshima	27.61×23.47	260	66.60	2.09±0.170	7,864
	27.54×23.81	640	44.54	0.324±0.0204	1,188
	27.30×23.89	779	41.69	0.146±0.0013	541
	27.50×46.12	1,180	27.65	0.0124±0.0023	51
Nagasaki	51.29×46.02	590	42.55	0.140±0.0066	514
	50.42×46.49	1,030	31.79	0.0127±0.0010	52

[a] The figures indicate the measured values in the summer of 1963.

TABLE III. Thermoluminescent Yield of Bricks and Tiles and Resultant Gamma Ray Dose (NIRS)

City	Coordinates of samples	Distance from ground zero (m)	Incident angle (°)	Luminescence L	Gamma ray dose (rad)
Hiroshima	27.37×23.53	140	79.46	21.4±1.4	10,118
	27.53×23.51	155	11.64	26.3±1.0	9,990
	27.36×23.43	170	73.44	20.4±1.1	8,578
	27.70×23.33	415	57.60	18.9±0.9	4,065
	27.84×23.45	605	45.41	24.0±1.2	1,582
	27.90×23.43	710	40.46	29.0±2.4	1,043
	27.43×23.45	965	34.76	38.8±2.3	338
Nagasaki	51.00×46.13	95	12.00	160.0±4.0	24,311
	51.23×46.29	520	46.75	213.0±6.0	6,435
	50.60×46.33	635	38.73	40.8±0.2	4,240
	50.39×46.22	860	31.69	11.8±1.1	1,639
	50.38×46.20	875	30.72	21.8±1.3	1,471
	51.23×45.68	970	27.65	12.0±1.0	937
	51.24×45.68	1,020	26.57	70.0±1.4	824

A) *Neutrons*

Cobalt is contained in iron as an impurity though in a very minute quantity. ^{59}Co is activated when irradiated by thermal neutrons and becomes ^{60}Co, which has a half-life of 5.27 years and emits beta rays with a maximum energy of 0.3 MeV. For the measurement of extremely weak activity of ^{60}Co, a coincidence type of beta ray spectrometer was used. In order to reduce the effect of self-absorption of beta rays on the activity measurement, the cobalt elements in iron samples were chemically separated and the Co fraction was deposited on a platinum planchet by electroplating.

Assuming that the spectrum of neutrons at distances greater than 500 m from ground zero was composed of a fast neutron component having a similar energy spectrum to that of the HPRR at ORNL, free-in-air neutron doses per unit specific activity of ^{60}Co were determined with an experiment in which iron rods imbedded in the concrete blocks at nearly 8 cm deep from the surface were irradiated with neutrons from the HPRR at ORNL. Table II gives the resultant specific activities and free-in-air neutron doses (*13*).

B) *Gamma rays*

When thermoluminescent materials are exposed to ionizing radiations, some of the free electrons are trapped at lattice imperfections in the crystalline solid. They remain trapped for long periods at ambient temperatures. If the temperature is increased, electrons are thermally released from the traps and light is emitted as they recombine with oppositely charged centers. The quantity of light emitted can be proportional to the absorbed energy in the material. Bricks and tiles can be utilized as thermoluminescent materials (*5*).

The thermoluminescent yield of bricks and ornamental tiles was measured with a handmade apparatus. The gamma ray dose of the A-bombs was estimated from the results of the thermoluminescent measurements, using a gamma ray source spectrally equivalent to the A-bombs prepared by X-rays from a 6 MeV linear accelerator for a high energy component and gamma rays from ^{60}Co and ^{137}Cs for a medium energy component. Table III gives the results of the thermoluminescent measurements and resultant free-in-air gamma ray doses (*15*).

C) Kyoto University

A group at Kyoto University (*15*) has estimated free-in-air gamma ray doses with thermoluminescent measurements of roof tiles.

6. *Free-in-air doses of T65D*

The precision (coefficient of variation) of NIRS dose estimates was estimated to be less than 0.11 for gamma rays and less than 0.15 for neutrons. NIRS doses as compared with York's values shown in Fig. 3 provided only a minor difference for gamma rays and agreed with that for neutrons in Nagasaki, but a large difference of approximately 50% for neutrons and 30%–70% for gamma rays at distances of 500–1,500 m from ground zero in Hiroshima. Auxier and his co-workers (*4*) estimated the percent probable error in their dose estimates. Because of the uncertainties which persist concerning the yield of the Hiroshima bomb, the error in the Hiroshima estimates was considered to be about 30%. The doses for Nagasaki were estimated to be accurate to within about 10%.

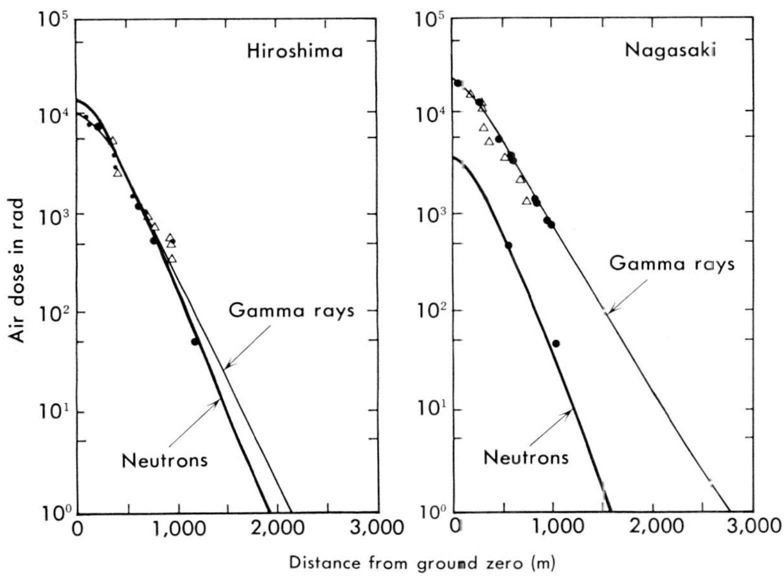

FIG. 4. T65D free-in-air doses for ORNL and Japanese data, Hiroshima and Nagasaki. ═, ORNL; •●, NIRS; △, Kyoto University.

The free-in-air doses of gamma rays and neutrons determined by *in situ* measurements by two Japanese groups agreed with the ORNL values estimated as a result of Operation BREN (Fig. 4), although there is some scatter. Milton and Shohoji (*24*) have described the T65D system of dose estimates in Hiroshima and Nagasaki. They proposed the free-in-air dose curves calculated from the parameters given by Auxier *et al.* (*4*) in the T65D system.

7. *Nine parameters*

Gamma rays and neutrons differ in their penetration, and shielding materials in their penetrability. For survivors in the open unshielded on all sides, the best estimates of the dose received are free-in-air doses. However, survivors shielded on one side by a heavy wall received the full free-in-air dose less some fraction screened out by the wall. The survivors exposed in a house received only a small fraction of the free-in-air dose at a corresponding distance, depending on numerous characteristics of the shielding configuration. The ORNL group developed a technique of globe operation to evaluate transmission values for these shielding situations. The globe consisted of a sphere of transparent plastic with latitude and longitude lines inscribed on the surface at 10° intervals and a small bulb approximating a point source of light at the center. When placed in a scale model of the shielding configuration so that its center represents the survivor of interest, the axis was pointed in the direction of the radiation source, and its projection on portions of the model showed what part of the incident radiation was intercepted by the shield. Using the experimentally determined angular distribution function of radiations from the A-bomb tests in conjunction with the measurements made with the globe operation, the fraction of intercepted radiations was determined. The dose at the point of interest, D, was calculated by the following equation:

$$D=(TF_1+F_2)D_{\mathrm{air}} \tag{2}$$

where F_1 is the fraction of radiation intercepted, T is the transmission rate of the shield, F_2 is the fraction of total radiation which is not blocked, and D_{air} is the free-in-air dose at the location.

In addition to the globe operation, the ORNL group developed a more sophisticated nine parameter procedure to estimate the transmission rates to be applied to the free-in-air dose for the evaluations of the dose for survivors exposed in typical Japanese houses. The nine parameters for gamma rays and neutrons were 1) floor number, 2) slant penetration distance of direct radiation through the house, 3) number of interior walls shielding the survivors from the front, 4) number of interior walls shielding the survivor from the side, 5) presence of a shielding structure in front, 6) size of the shielding structure in front, if present, 7) presence of a lateral shielding structure, 8) distance from any unshielded window in the direction of the burst point, and 9) height above the air/ground interface. Using these parameters, the radiation dose at the point of interest was calculated by the following equation:

Neutrons:

$$D_n=[A_1\exp(-G_1)+A_2G_2+A_3G_3+A_4G_4+A_5G_5+A_6\exp(-G_6)+A_8G_8+A_8]D_{\mathrm{air}} \tag{3}$$

Gamma rays:

$$D_\gamma=[A_1A_2\exp(-G)+A_2\exp(-G_1)+A_4G_3+A_5G_4+A_6G_5+A_7G_6]D_{\mathrm{air}} \tag{4}$$

TABLE IV. BREN Average Gamma Ray Transmission Factors for a Single-story House in Hiroshima

Event	Neutron	Gamma ray
Plumbbob	0.507 ± 0.11	0.769 ± 0.11
Hardtack	0.407 ± 0.09	0.952 ± 0.15
BREN reactor	0.151 ± 0.15	1.35 ± 0.08
BREN ^{60}Co		0.464 ± 0.18

where D_n represents neutron dose and D_γ gamma ray dose in Japanese houses or other structures. A_i is the constant and G_i is a geometrical factor related to the nine parameters. The ratios of D_n/D_{air} and D_γ/D_{air} represent the transmission factor for neutrons and gamma rays, respectively. The BREN average gamma ray transmission factors for a single house at Hiroshima and Nagasaki are given in Table IV. These numbers are based on the single house experiment with the HPRR and ^{60}Co gamma ray source. The effect of surrounding houses on the transmission factor (*1*) was assumed to change the single house value by a power of 2 and 3/2, respectively.

In the dose determinations for survivors in the LSS, organ or tissue doses should be evaluated using the house transmission factors and dose distributions of A-bomb radiation in the body of the survivor. The NIRS and ORNL groups have determined some conversion factors from free-in-air doses to organ or tissue doses for the organ dosimetry (*9–12*, *16*).

To evaluate the late biological effects of the A-bombs a primary requirement is the most precise knowledge concerning not only the exposure to the initial radiations of the bombs but the exposure to secondary radiations from residual radiations released from neutron-induced radioactivity and fission products on the ground and medical exposure before and after the time of bombs. The latter doses have been evaluated by some authors (*8*, *25*, *33*).

Recent Reassessments of A-Bomb Radiation Dosimetry

There are significant differences in the biological effects on the survivors in Hiroshima and Nagasaki. In the T65D system, these differences appeared to be explained by the existence of a significant neutron dose in Hiroshima as compared with the dose in Nagasaki. Milton and Shohoji (*24*) predicted that the T65D estimates were not final and should be revised immediately when new information became available. A-bomb dose depends on many factors, such as the design of the bomb, the TNT equivalent yield, the height above the ground at which the bomb explodes, the density and humidity of the air, and numerous other factors. Information on source terms such as spectra and intensities of radiation sources is very important for the dose estimations of survivors after an explosion of an A-bomb and even after a critical accident in nuclear facilities.

The first modern calculations of the output spectra of neutrons and gamma rays from the A-bombs exploded over Hiroshima and Nagasaki were declassified by the US Department of Energy (DOE) in 1976 and were distributed as a letter (*36*) which was used in recent reassessments of A-bomb doses. The ORNL (*17*) and LLNL (*20*) groups recalculated the free-in-air doses of gamma rays and neutrons on the basis of the output spectra calculated by Preeg, using a computer code employing "discrete ordinate transport" (DOT) techniques. Components on which they recalculated the dose

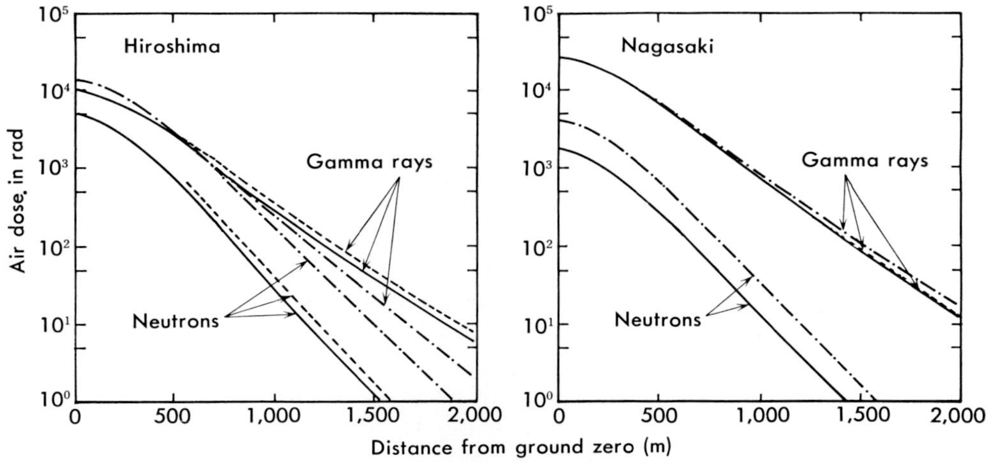

FIG. 5. Revised free-in-air doses by ORNL (*17*) and LLNL (*20*), Hiroshima and Nagasaki. -·-, T65D; ——, ORNL; ----, LLNL.

TABLE V. Differences of Dose Determination between LLNL and ORNL

Parameter	LLNL	ORNL
Source terms	Preeg-LANL	Preeg-LANL
Transport calculation	DOT technique-ORNL	DOT technique-ORNL
Cross-section	ENDL	ENDF/B-IV and V
Atmosphere (ground-burst height)	Homogeneous	Tiered with decreasing density of air with height
Ground composition	4 elements (H, O, Si, and Al)	(H, O, Si, and Al)
Height of burst	Hiroshima, 570 m Nagasaki, 503 m	Hiroshima, 580 m Nagasaki, 503 m
Yield of bomb	Hiroshima, 15 kton Nagasaki, 22 kton	Hiroshima, 12.5 kton Nagasaki, 22 kton
Delayed gamma ray calculation code	ITTRI (1964) (semi-experimental)	NUIDEA (1981) (theoretical)

consisted of 1) prompt gamma rays and neutrons from bomb leakage directly out of the weapon, 2) secondary component of gamma rays resulting from neutron interactions with atmospheric nitrogen, and 3) gamma rays from the debris cloud of a nuclear explosion. Their results are shown in Fig. 5. The data do not completely agree with each other because they used some different factors and some different assumptions in their dose calculations (Table V). As shown in Fig. 5, the neutron dose in Hiroshima was much less than the T65D estimates by factors varying from about 4 at a ground distance of 1,000 m to 8 at 2,000 m, and the gamma ray doses were greater than the T65D estimates starting at a ground distance of about 1,000 m and were probably larger by a factor of about 3 at 2,000 m. In Nagasaki, the situation was reversed with respect to gamma rays, and the T65D estimates were higher, but the differences were small, for example, about 20% at a ground distance of 1,000 m and 30% at 2,000 m. Although these results are preliminary, the T65D estimates must be revised on the basis of new information such as leakage output radiation spectra from the A-bombs.

The neutron and gamma ray doses received by the survivors in Hiroshima and Nagasaki must be accurate within some limits if conclusions drawn from studies of the survivors are to be of value. The accuracy of each factor related to the dose assessments must be shown by comparing the calculated data with observed data from the A-bomb tests in Nevada and other pertinent experiments as well as with physical data from *in situ* measurements such as sulphur and cobalt activations at Hiroshima and Nagasaki. Furthermore, to reanalyze data on observed biological effects in the survivors, some dosimetric factors should be investigated in more detail.

1. Yields of Hiroshima and Nagasaki explosions

The yield of the A-bombs is extremely important for estimations of the source terms. The yields of the Nagasaki bomb and Hiroshima bomb were estimated to be 22 ktons and 12.5 ktons, respectively, in the previous T65D dose determinations. The current yield of the Nagasaki bomb has been well established by radiochemical and fireball data obtained from tests at Nevada, together with calculations, as 22±2 ktons. The Hiroshima bomb yield has been determined by comparison with similar effects at Nagasaki. Malik (*21*) determined a yield of 12±4 ktons for blast effects and 15±3 ktons for thermal effects in Hiroshima. Tajima (*32*) reevaluated recently the Hiroshima yield as about 14 ktons from a measurement of the thermal effect on Japanese cypress board exposed to the A-bomb in Hiroshima. The recent best yield estimate for Hiroshima is 15±3 ktons (*39*).

2. Source terms of initial radiations

Whalen (*37*) reconfirmed the validity of the output spectra obtained by one-dimensional calculations. The spherical model of the bomb was a good approximation for the Nagasaki-type weapon. The Hiroshima bomb was a very nonspherical construction. Whalen and his co-workers determined a Hiroshima bomb spectrum with two-dimensional calculations. The neutron spectrum for the Hiroshima bomb from the Preeg one-dimensional calculation is compared with the result from the Whalen two-dimensional calculation (*37*) in Fig. 6. In the approximately cylindrical Hiroshima bomb, the two-dimensional effects reduce the neutron output by 16% from the spherical calculation. The neutron dose is reduced by 21%. The results of one- and two-dimensional calculations for the gamma ray output spectra of the Hiroshima bomb are shown in Fig. 7.

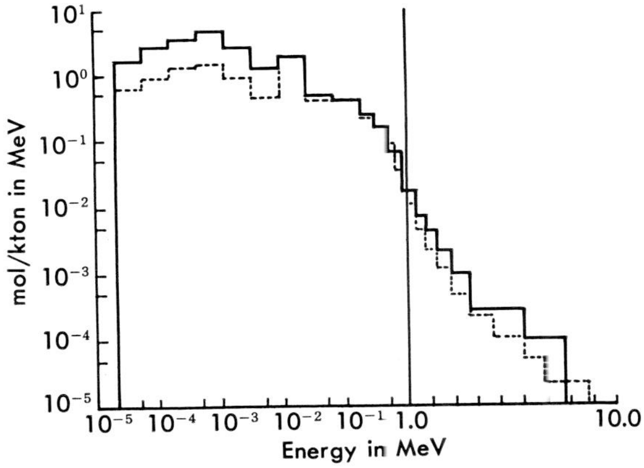

FIG. 6. Neutron spectra for the Hiroshima-type bomb. ——, Preeg; ----, two-dimensional.

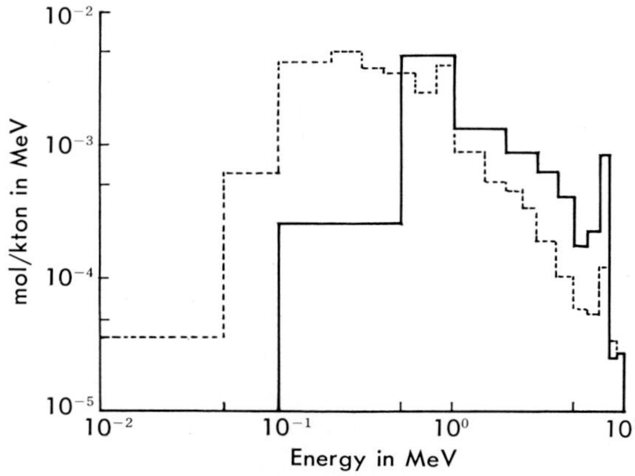

FIG. 7. Gamma ray spectra for the Hiroshima-type bomb. ——, Preeg; ----, two-dimensional.

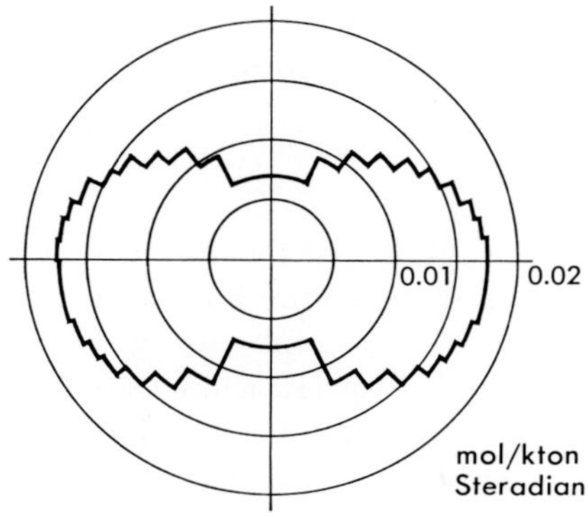

FIG. 8. Angular distribution of neutrons from the Hiroshima bomb.

The calculated output gamma ray energy is greatly reduced in the two-dimensional calculation, going from the one-dimensional value of 0.019 MeV mol per kiloton to the two-dimensional value of 0.007 MeV mol per kiloton (*37*). The results of the two-dimensional calculations were confirmed with a spectral measurement using fissionable material which was raised into the center of the Hiroshima-type bomb assembly. Whalen has also suggested that the Hiroshima bomb had the strong angular distributions of neutrons as shown in Fig. 8.

3. Air-transport calculations

The output spectrum of neutrons more than 1 keV had average energy of about 1.6 MeV for the Nagasaki-type bomb and only about 0.3 MeV for the Hiroshima bomb (*18*). Only a small fraction of the neutrons escaped from the Nagasaki bomb as fast neutrons, but these were quite energetic because of hardening of the neutron spectrum by the hydrogen content in the thick charges of high explosive. Mostly fast neutrons escaped from the Hiroshima bomb, but they were severely degraded in energy because of softening of the neutron spectrum by the iron and other heavy materials in the massive bomb casing (*27*).

TABLE VI. Comparison of Air Density and Atmosphere Water Vapor Content at Explosion, Hiroshima and Nagasaki

	Hiroshima			Nagasaki		
	JWA	Kerr *et al.*	Δ (%)	JWA	Kerr *et al.*	Δ (%)
Relative humidity (%)						
Ground level	80	80		71	71	
Burst height	84	75	10.7	71	67	5.6
Moist air density (kg/m³)						
Ground level	1.203	1.170	2.7	1.192	1.158	2.9
Burst height	1.139	1.110	2.5	1.138	1.106	2.8
Dry air density (kg/m³)						
Ground level	1.184	1.150	2.9	1.172	1.137	3.0
Burst height	1.122	1.094	2.5	1.122	1.090	2.9
Absolute humidity (kg/m³)						
Ground level	0.0203	0.02025	—	0.0202	0.0202	—
Burst height	0.01720	0.01564	9.0	0.01610	0.01613	0.0
Mean density (kg/m³)						
Moist air	1.171	1.140	2.6	1.165	1.132	2.8
Dry air	1.152	1.122	2.6	1.147	1.114	2.9
Water vapor	0.01869	0.1785	4.0	0.01817	0.01808	0.5

JWA: Japan Weather Association.

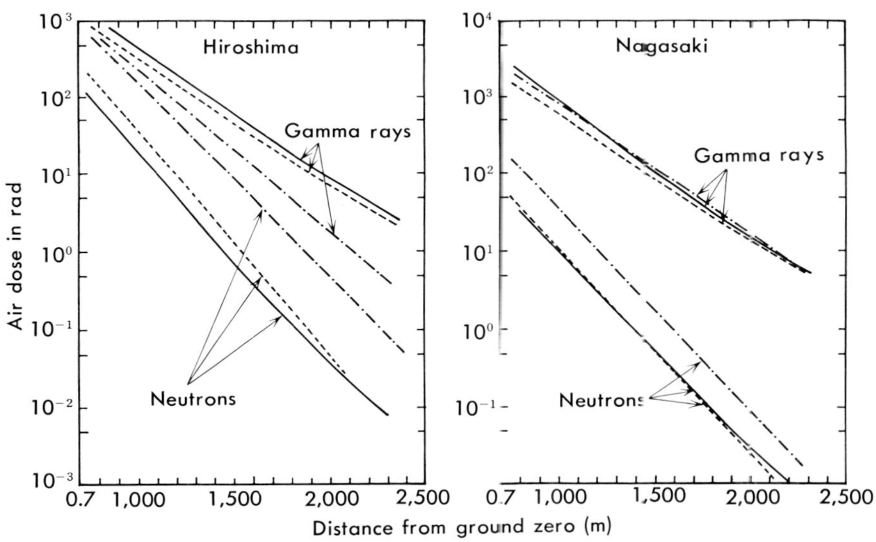

FIG. 9. Recently revised free-in-air doses by ORNL and LLNL, Hiroshima and Nagasaki. -·-, T65D; ——, ORNL and SAI; ----, LLNL.

Fast neutrons from the A-bombs lose their kinetic energy in air mostly through elastic collision with the hydrogen elements in moisture. Consequently, the moisture content of air is an important parameter for the calculations of neutrons in air. The T65D has been determined principally by BREN measurements in dry air at the Nevada Test Site. However, the relative humidity at the time of the explosions in Hiroshima and Nagasaki (*32*) was very high as given in Table VI. Kerr (*17*) and Loewe and Mendelsohn (*20*) have calculated the free-in-air neutron dose, taking into account the high humidity in both cities as given in Table V. Kerr carried out the dose calculations assuming layered moist air having an exponentially decreasing density between the ground and the burst height of the bomb. There was no significant discrepancy between the estimates of atmospheric conditions by Kerr (*17*) and by RERF (32).

Recently, Kerr *et al.* (*19*) have been calculating the free-in-air doses in an air-over-ground geometry from prompt gamma rays and neutrons and from secondary gamma rays produced in air and in soil by the interaction with neutrons, using the two-dimensional DOT-IV code developed by ORNL and recently calculated source terms by Whalen. Also, they have been calculating the free-in-air doses at ground level from delayed gamma rays and delayed neutrons, using the NUIDEA code developed by Scott (*29*). Figure 9 shows the recent data on the free-in-air doses in Hiroshima and Nagasaki.

4. *Delayed radiation*

Gamma rays from the debris cloud of the explosion contributed a considerable fraction of the total free-in-air gamma ray dose on the ground at long distances from ground zero in Hiroshima and Nagasaki. The delayed gamma rays were received in the first about 10 sec after the explosion, before the rising fireball carried fission products away from the ground. The time dependency of the delayed gamma ray doses is complicated by various factors such as air shock in the amount of air between the source and a point of interest on the ground and the fission product decay rate. The time-dependent measurements of the gamma ray dose rate had been carried out previously for various yields and burst heights during the Nevada tests. Several calculation models of delayed gamma ray dose were examined and compared with the results of the A-bomb tests. Scott (*29*) developed the NUIDEA model which incorporated the most detailed hydrodynamic and fireball model. Loewe and Mendelsohn (*20*) used the ITTRI model for the calculation of delayed gamma rays. Since the delayed gamma ray radiations from the decay of fission products in the fireball account for 40%–60% of the total gamma ray dose in Hiroshima and Nagasaki, the uncertainty in the determination of fission-product dose should be reduced as low as reasonably achievable.

5. *In situ measurements in Japan*

Recent dose estimations of the A-bombs in Hiroshima and Nagasaki have been carried out only with calculations, using a large computer. Information obtained from some experimental values of physical or chemical changes in materials exposed to the A-bombs in Hiroshima and Nagasaki is primarily important for the dose estimations. These *in situ* measurements hold the key to dose reevaluation of the Hiroshima and Nagasaki A-bombs.

A) *Sulphur activation*

On the day following each of the nuclear explosions, Japanese teams surveyed residual radioactivity at various sites in Hiroshima and Nagasaki. Yamazaki and Sugimoto (*42*) measured the radioactivity of ^{32}P produced by the reaction $^{32}S(n,p)^{32}P$ in sulphur used in utility pole insulators in Hiroshima. This reaction is caused by fast neutrons with energies above 2.5 MeV. Fast neutrons contribute predominantly to the total neutron dose. Therefore, the sulfur activations are important parameters for the estimation of energy spectrum and angular distributions, as well as for the dose estimations. The ORNL and SAI groups have been calculating ^{32}P activity in the utility

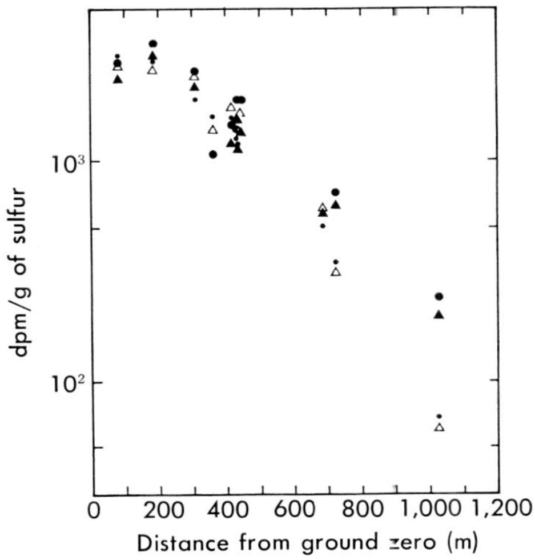

FIG. 10. Comparison between calculated and measured ^{32}P specific activities in sulfur materials, Hiroshima. ●, Yamasaki (1958); •, Pace and Kerr (BH270 tilt angle 0°); △, Pace and Kerr (BH270 tilt angle 15°); ▲, Yamasaki/Hamada (1983).

pole insulators to confirm the validity of their air-transport calculations by comparing the calculated values with the measured values. The differences in the ^{32}P activities measured at various sites were extremely important to determine the angle with respect to the vertical at the time of explosion of the Hiroshima bomb.

Recently, Hamada (*7*) of the Japan Radioisotope Association (JRIA) revised the values of ^{32}P activities measured by Yamasaki and Sugimoto (*42*) in 1945, using a Lauritsen electroscope and a uranium oxide (U_3O_8) beta ray source which Yamasaki used. The ORNL and SAI groups have been calculating ^{32}P activities in sulphur insulators taking account of the angular distribution of neutrons as shown in Fig. 8. Their preliminary results appear to explain successfully the results of ^{32}P activities revised by Hamada (*7*) as shown in Fig. 10 (*31*).

B) *Cobalt activation*

Hashizume *et al.* (*13*) had measured ^{60}Co activities produced in the 8 cm deep embedded iron sample by thermalization of fast neutrons within the concrete walls of buildings to evaluate free-in-air neutron doses from the activities. Since, however, the neutron spectrum which they used for the determination of conversion factors from activity to neutron dose was different from the recently calculated spectrum, the ORNL and LLNL groups suggested that the neutron doses estimated from the ^{60}Co activities should be revised. The LLNL group has calculated the ^{60}Co activities at various distances from ground zero with new techniques and cross-section data which they used for the reevaluation of doses in Hiroshima and Nagasaki. They have not yet obtained results which are in good agreement with the measured values, with the exception of the data at 1,180 m in Hiroshima (*20*).

C) *Thermoluminescent measurements*

Hashizume *et al.* (*13*) and Ichikawa *et al.* (*15*) previously used the thermoluminescent yields from bricks, ornamental tiles, and roof tiles to estimate the A-bomb doses in Hiroshima and Nagasaki. The recent estimates of gamma ray doses by the ORNL and

Alamos National Laboratory with the Replica of Hiroshima Weapon, Proc. 2nd A-bomb Dosimetry Workshop, Hiroshima, pp. 21–15 (1983).
39. Woolson, W. A. personal communication (1984).
40. Woolson, W. A. Gritzner, M. L., and Egbert, S. D. Coupled houseman shielding calculations for atomic bomb survivors organ dosimetry, Proc. Workshop, 2nd A-bomb Dosimetry Workshop, Hiroshima, pp. 72–75 (1982).
41. Woolson, W. A., Marcum, J., Scott, W. H., and Staggs, V. E. Building transmission factors, Proc. Symp. at Germantown, Technical Information Center US Department of Energy, pp. 179–208 (1982).
42. Yamazaki, F. and Sugimoto, A. Radioactive phosphorous ^{32}P in human bone and sulfur insulators in Hiroshima, Collection of Investigative Reports on Atomic Bomb Disaster, Vol. I, pp. 16–18 (1953). Japanese Science Promotion Society, Tokyo.

GANN Monograph on Cancer Research 32, 1986

TUMOR AND TISSUE REGISTRIES IN HIROSHIMA AND NAGASAKI

Tetsuo MONZEN[*1] and Toshiro WAKABAYASHI[*2]
Department of Pathology, Hiroshima Prefectural Hospital,[*1] *and Department of Epidemiology and Statistics*[*2], *Radiation Effects Research Foundation*

Continued monitoring of tumor incidence is an important part of the surveillance of health effects of atomic bomb (A-bomb) radiation. The Radiation Effects Research Foundation (RERF) (formerly Atomic Bomb Casualty Commission (ABCC)) has been engaged in the operation of tumor and tissue registries in Hiroshima and Nagasaki These registries have been instrumental in studying risk of various specific cancer sites (thyroid, breast, lung, stomach, colorectal, and salivary gland) in a defined sample of A-bomb survivors. A recent analysis of registry data revealed little basis for suspecting systematic biases of registry data (*e.g.*, hospital-related, or diagnostic biases related to radiation dose) which may confound observed association of cancer and radiation. The analysis also showed similarities in relative risk of cancer based on incidence and mortality data. However, absolute risks estimated from mortality data may underestimate the true magnitude for certain cancer sites (including breast, stomach, lung, and uterus). The registry data are also useful in assessing secular trends of radiation-induced cancer incidence which are essential in determining the latency of cancer.

The Atomic Bomb Casualty Commission (ABCC) and its successor, the Radiation Effects Research Foundation (RERF), have been engaged in the operation of tumor registries for the last 20 years and tissue registries for the last 10 years in Hiroshima and Nagasaki under the entrustment of local medical associations. These registries have served as important data sources in assessment of cancer incidence in the RERF sample of persons exposed to atomic bomb (A-bomb) radiation as well as geographically defined populations. Incidence data offer an advantage over mortality data in that the former provide a direct measure of cancer risk. This is particularly important when dealing with tumors associated with relatively low mortality such as thyroid and breast cancer. Also, detailed diagnostic information gathered from medical records can enhance accuracy of diagnosis. The significance of detailed diagnostic information is increased with the recent decline in autopsy rates.

Activities of the tumor registries in the early years were described in several publications (*5*, *6*, *8*). Later the tumor and tissue registry data have been used extensively at RERF for epidemiologic and pathologic studies of specific cancer cites in relation to A-bomb radiation exposure. These sites include thyroid, breast, lung, stomach, colorectal,

[*1] Ujina Kanda 1-5, Minami-ku, Hiroshima 730, Japan (門前徹夫).
[*2] Hijiyama Park 5-2, Minami-ku, Hiroshima 732, Japan (若林俊郎).

and salivary gland (*2, 12–14, 16, 18, 19, 22, 23*). Overall analysis of the latest tumor incidence data of the Life Span Study (LSS) sample in Nagasaki (for the period 1959–78) has been published (*17*). Recently analysis has been made of the updated Hiroshima registry data and the findings of this analysis are to be published.

Tumor Registry

Agreements were exchanged between ABCC and the City Medical Associations of Hiroshima and Nagasaki for the initiation of Tumor Registries in Hiroshima in 1957 and in Nagasaki in 1958. The City Medical Associations of the two cities have organized the Tumor Statistics Committee which is responsible for the maintenance of the Registry and registration of tumor cases, while ABCC (and later RERF) provided technical support. At the outset, registration was quite active as described in several reports (*5, 6, 8*). It became less active in subsequent years, especially in Hiroshima, mainly because of difficulty in securing collaboration from large hospitals. However, through concentrated efforts during the past few years in updating data collection, the Hiroshima registry data now appear to merit analysis.

For registries to be effective, all tumor cases should be ascertained. While cases with histologically confirmed neoplasms are ideal for diagnostic accuracy, they may represent a small and possibly selected portion of tumor cases. The Hiroshima and Nagasaki registries, like most other registries, assemble information from various data sources (clinical, pathological, radiological, *etc.*).

As a rule the examining physician is requested to submit a report whenever a case is detected. A notification card in a sealed envelope is used for preservation of confidentiality and privacy. Major hospitals are also requested to submit their reports once a month. As the burden of assigned physicians at these major hospitals is heavy, and the assignment is often rotated among the physicians, the number of reports submitted is not always constant. Cases reported by physicians (private or at hospitals) make up only a small proportion of all registered patients (10% in Hiroshima and 3% in Nagasaki).

Most cases (79% in Hiroshima and 85% in Nagasaki) are ascertained by screening of hospitalized tumor cases undertaken by trained RERF field personnel. They search autopsy protocols, clinical and pathological reports, as well as surgical operation records. At surgery, tumors can be confirmed directly, and with recent progress in operative techniques, surgical records are an especially useful source of data on nonfatal cancers (*e.g.*, breast, uterine cervix, and urinary bladder). X-ray diagnoses and clinical examinations are still important sources of data, and diagnosis by cytologic and endoscopic examination has recently increased. The latter should be classified separately, but the number of cases is still small and therefore is included in the clinical diagnosis category. When information obtained from these various sources is checked against death certificates, many tumors are found for which no hospital record has been obtained. Thus, death certificates remain an important source of ascertainment, accounting for 11% of all cases in Hiroshima and 12% in Nagasaki.

Registered tumors are all malignant neoplasms plus benign neoplasms of the brain, salivary gland, and colon. Polyposis of the stomach and digestive organs is also included. Information is gathered on name, sex, date of birth, present address, tumor diagnosed, method and date of diagnosis, date of death and medical institution, and clinic or physician. Information obtained is checked against the Master File to determine whether it

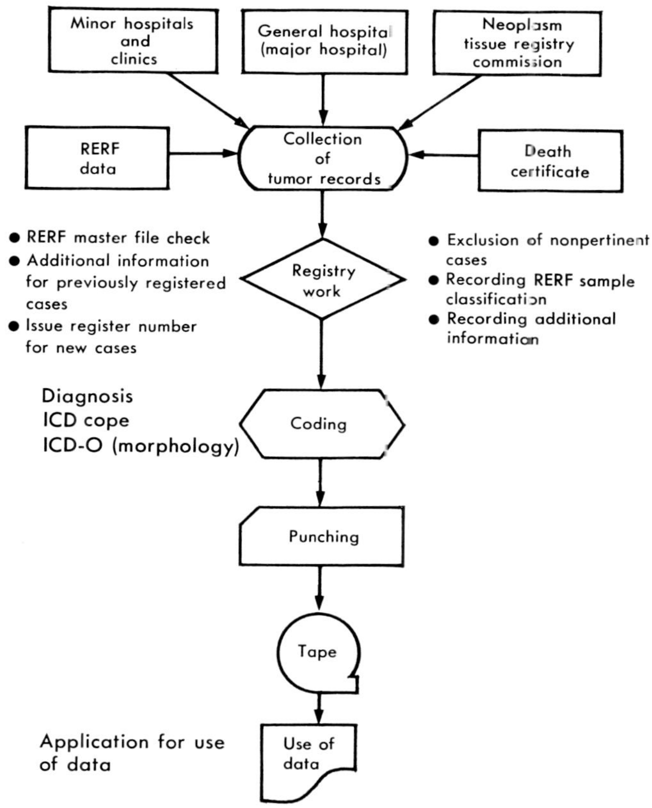

FIG. 1. Flow chart, Tumor Registry.

is a new or registered case. After determining the validity of registration, a code is assigned based on the International Classification of Diseases (ICD) 9th revision (*21*) and the data are stored on magnetic tapes (Fig. 1).

Multiple reports of the same tumor sometimes occur. There are cases in which the same cancer is reported by different hospitals, at different periods, with diagnosis based on different diagnostic methods. When this occurs, a report using the best available information is coded and filed. Among the alternative methods of ascertainment, autopsy findings take precedence followed by surgical pathological statements, surgical findings, radiography, clinical examinations, and finally the statement as to cause of death recorded on the death certificate.

Among the clinically diagnosed cases are those which the attending physician labeled possible cancer (*e.g.*, possible cancer of the stomach or possible pancreatic cancer). The qualification "possible" is maintained in the computer record so that analysis can be made excluding these cases, if desired. It has been suggested that overregistration may have occurred due to inclusion of possible cancer and occult cancer (recognized only at autopsy) in the Hiroshima and Nagasaki data. The proportion of possible cancer cases among total cases is 8.6% in Hiroshima and 12.6% in Nagasaki. They are relatively less frequent in Hiroshima than in Nagasaki and their contribution to over-registration is less in Hiroshima. The mean frequency of autopsy among deaths occurring in the LSS sample during 1961–75, which is the major source of detecting occult cancer, is 31%

in Hiroshima and 30% in Nagasaki, so it is likely that occult cancer influences the two registries in a similar way.

If a patient is registered with multiple tumor sites, it is difficult to determine whether they are single or multiple primary tumors, particularly on the basis of the limited clinical and pathologic information available. In our tumor registries, multiple cancers are registered whenever a case of multiple primary cancer is suspected, and such cases are reviewed using the guidelines on cancer registration published by the International Agency for Research on Cancer (*11*). In Hiroshima 204 (3%) of 6,608 reviewed cases were considered to have multiple primary cancer and in Nagasaki, 46 (2%) of 1,870 cases were regarded as multiple primary cancer.

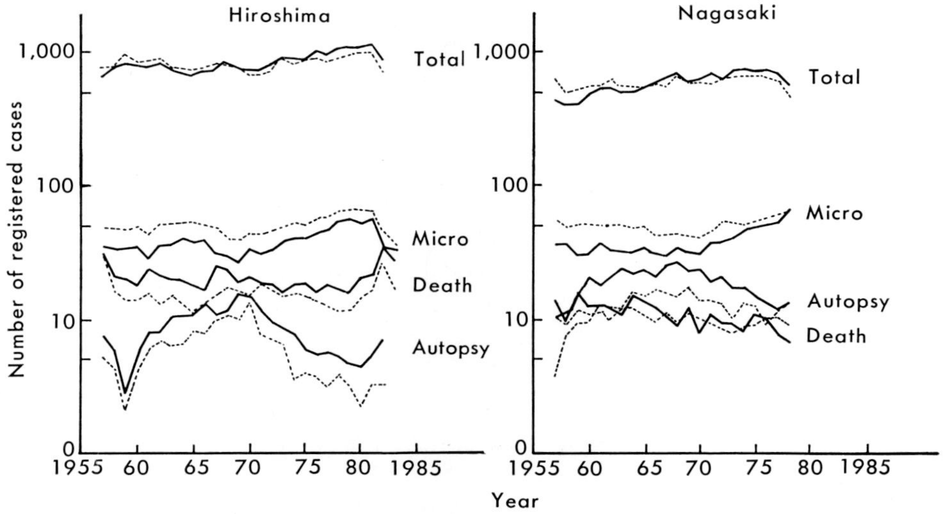

FIG. 2. Tumor Registry activities by city, sex, and year. Total number of registered cases. Rates for autopsies, microscopically confirmed cases, and death certificate only cases. ——, male; ----, female.

TABLE I. Average Annual Incidence Rate (per 100,000) in Hiroshima City, Nagasaki City, and Japan

City	Sex	Year		
		1975–77	1976–78	1977–79
Hiroshima	Male	223.6	236.5	239.6
	Female	164.6	162.2	162.3
Nagasaki	Male	250.4	252.6	257.6
	Female	184.6	178.8	175.9
		1976	1977	1978
Japan (estimates)	Male	203.3	206.1	209.4
	Female	136.0	137.9	138.5

Age-adjusted to world population.

Estimated incidence for Japan is obtained from Cancer Incidence in Japan 1975–79 (*4*). Hiroshima incidence rates are based on RERF's most recent estimates.

Data are routinely tabulated by site, age, and hospital, and the tabulations are distributed to each cooperative hospital in Hiroshima as feedback material. Stored information has been used at RERF for studies of several specific cancer sites. Comparative incidence studies among several tumor registries have also been conducted in cooperation with the cancer research group based on research funds from the Ministry of Health and Welfare.

Figure 2 presents the registered cases over the years in Hiroshima and Nagasaki by different ascertainment methods. The proportion of cases identified from death certificates alone has been relatively low, especially in Nagasaki. Table I shows the cancer incidence rate generated from the Hiroshima and Nagasaki registry data. Compared with the average cancer incidence rate for other prefectural registries in Japan, the age-adjusted incidence rates for all sites in both Hiroshima and Nagasaki are slightly higher. Several reasons for this are possible, including 1) the completeness of reports resulting from active data collection utilizing field personnel as compared to voluntary reporting by other registries; 2) overregistration because of the inclusion of doubtful diagnosis and occult cancer in the Hiroshima and Nagasaki registries; and 3) the high incidence of cancer in Hiroshima and Nagasaki.

Tissue Registry

In 1973, the Hiroshima Prefectural Medical Association initiated a Tissue Registry for registering surgical and pathological specimens of tumor tissues. The significance of this program lies in the collection of tumor cases based on tissue diagnosis and their reproducibility. Financial support was provided for three years from the US National Institutes of Health-National Cancer Institute to the Hiroshima Prefectural Medical Association *via* ABCC. With this support, the Medical Association organized the Hiroshima Prefectural Tissue Registry Committee and established its Registration Office at the Medical Association Hall. The registry is operated by a working committee composed of pathologists engaged in histological diagnosis at principal medical institutions, epidemiologists, statisticians, and representatives from the Leukemia Registry.

The Registration Office headed by an experienced pathologist requests the pathologist-in-charge at each medical institution to submit one H & E-stained tissue slide, a copy of the pathological diagnosis made at the institution, and a copy of the pathology examination request forwarded from clinical departments. For each reported case, a part-time pathologist reviews slides and assigns ICD-Oncology Codes (*20*).

In Hiroshima, approximately 14,000 tissue slides are submitted yearly, and approximately 10,000 cases are finally registered. The ratio of malignant cases to benign cases is about 3 to 2. In males, this ratio is 3 to 1, but it is higher in females due to benign tumors of the uterus, ovary, and breast.

The Tissue Registry in Nagasaki was begun in 1974, a year after the initiation of the Hiroshima Tissue Registry. Funding and establishment conditions were similar to those in Hiroshima. The Nagasaki Tissue Registry is conducted by the City Medical Association, which organized the Nagasaki Neoplasm Tissue Registry Commission and established the Registration Office in the Department of Pathology, Nagasaki University School of Medicine. The geographic area covered includes Nagasaki City and three adjacent cities and their suburbs. Different from the Hiroshima registry, tissue blocks are collected along with brief clinical records. Four specimens are prepared from each block at the Tissue Registry Laboratory and they are reviewed by four pathologists on the Pathology Expert Committee. If an agreement cannot be reached on diagnosis, the slides are submitted for review at a later date. The Manual of Tumor Nomenclature and Coding is employed for coding (*1*).

Analysis of Incidence Data

Data accumulated in the Tumor Registries have been found invaluable in assessing the carcinogenic role of radiation. Almost all of the original data for RERF cancer studies (including thyroid, breast, lung, stomach, colorectal, and salivary gland) are based on data from the Tumor and Tissue Registries. Overall analysis of Tumor Registry data in both cities has recently been completed for the period 1959–78, and some of the findings from this analysis are presented.

Subjects included in the analysis are members of the LSS extended sample in Nagasaki and alive as of January 1959. There are 17,936 persons in the sample, constituting a total of 319,803 person-years at risk during the observation period 1959–78. The dosimetry used is based on a revision of the original T65 dose system (T65DR), which takes into account the recently relocated Nagasaki ground zero point (*10*) and a standardization of the rounding process in calculating individual dose (*15*).

1. Potential sources of bias

Several potential sources of bias in the registry data may lead to spuriously increased cancer incidence in high radiation dose groups compared with low radiation or control groups. For example, biases related to radiation dose may originate in hospitals from which registry data were obtained. However, the distribution of registered tumor

TABLE II. Number of All Cancer Sites by Hospital and Exposure Status, Nagasaki, 1959–78

Hospital	T65 revised kerma dose in rad						NIC[a]	Unknown
	Total	0	1–9	10–49	50–99	100+		
Total	1,412	274	455	262	107	314	404	54
	100.0%	19.4%	32.2%	18.6%	7.6%	22.2%		
ABCC/RERF	520	103	153	96	45	123	156	20
	100.0	19.8	29.4	18.5	8.6	23.7		
Nagasaki University	347	61	116	61	28	81	91	18
	100.0	17.6	33.4	17.6	8.1	23.3		
Citizens hospital	78	17	25	17	5	14	35	2
	100.0	21.8	32.1	21.8	6.4	17.9		
A-bomb hospital	207	40	73	36	9	49	19	8
	100.0	19.3	35.3	17.4	4.3	23.7		
Other large hospitals	128	28	36	28	11	25	35	4
	100.0	21.9	28.1	21.9	8.6	19.5		
Practitioners (private)	79	13	32	16	7	11	35	2
	100.0	16.5	40.5	20.2	8.9	13.9		
Other	53	12	20	8	2	11	33	0
	100.0	22.6	37.7	15.1	3.8	20.8		

[a] Not in the city.

Difference in distribution by hospital among five exposed groups (NIC and Unknown excluded). Not significant. $\chi^2=18.46$, $d.f.=24$, $p=0.78$.

TABLE III. Number of All Cancer Sites by Method of Ascertainment and Exposure Status, Nagasaki, 1959–78

	T65 revised kerma dose in rad						NIC[a]	Unknown
	Total	0	1–9	10–49	50–99	100+		
Total	1,412	274	455	262	107	314	404	54
	100.0%	100.0%	100.0%	100.0%	100.0%	100.0%		
a) Confirmed	1,015	186	335	188	85	221	273	37
	71.9	67.9	73.6	71.8	79.4	70.4		
1. Autopsy	420	76	140	82	40	82	114	19
	29.7	27.8	30.8	31.3	37.4	26.1		
2. Surgical	514	96	164	89	36	129	136	15
	36.4	35.0	36.0	34.0	33.6	41.1		
3. Operation	81	14	31	17	9	10	23	3
	5.7	5.1	6.8	6.5	8.4	3.2		
b) Other	397	88	120	74	22	93	131	17
	28.1	32.1	26.4	28.2	20.6	29.6		
4. Radiography	129	34	37	25	6	27	35	7
	9.1	12.4	8.1	9.5	5.6	8.6		
5. Clinical	173	36	48	32	9	48	42	8
	12.3	13.1	10.6	12.2	8.4	15.3		
6. Death certificate	95	18	35	17	7	18	54	2
	6.7	6.6	7.7	6.5	6.6	5.7		

[a] Not in the city.

Difference in distribution by six methods of ascertainment is not significant among five exposure groups (NIC and Unknown excluded). $\chi^2=24.54$, $d.f.=20$, $p=0.22$.

Difference in distribution by Confirmed and Other is not significant among five exposure groups (NIC and Unknown excluded). $\chi^2=6.2$, $d.f.=4$, $p=0.18$.

cases by radiation dose did not differ among hospitals (Table II). Knowledge of dose on the part of the physician and/or survivor may result in frequent use of certain diagnostic techniques (*e.g.*, surgical pathology) or infrequent use of other methods (*e.g.*, radiography) among A-bomb survivors. However, data in Table III show no consistent pattern for preferred diagnostic methods by dose group. The highest dose group (100+ rad) had fewer cases undergoing autopsy and more cases subjected to pathologic examination, but the difference was not statistically significant. Cases confirmed by autopsy, surgical pathology, or surgery accounted for 72% of all cases, and the proportion of confirmed cases did not differ by dose group. Based on these findings there is little evidence to suspect the presence of systematic biases in the registry data.

Another source of potential bias is differential migration for different dose groups. Separate analysis of data from a subset of the LSS failed to disclose differential rates of migration for various dose groups or by time period (*3*). More recently, other evidence on this issue has become available as a result of a mail survey of exposed LSS members. These data, too, fail to reveal systematic differences in migration by dose and time which could obscure a radiation effect on cancer incidence or create a spurious one.

2. *Cancer risk and radiation exposure*

Table IV presents the relative risk for all and selected sites of cancer for the 100+ rad group (*vs.* 0–9 or 0 rad groups), using three sources of ascertainment: all sources (all); autopsy, pathology, and surgery reports (confirmed); and death certificates (mor-

TABLE IV. Relative Risk (100+ *vs.* 0–9 rad) of All and Selected Cancer by Method of Ascertainment: Nagasaki, 1959–78

Site	Source		
	All sources	Confirmed	Mortality
All sites[a]	1.70 (1.48 1.95)	1.76 (1.49 2.07)	1.29 (1.05 1.56)
Leukemia	3.49 (1.47 7.65)	3.49 (1.47 7.65)	3.73 (1.57 8.19)
All except leukemia[a]	1.67 (1.46 1.92)	1.72 (1.46 2.03)	1.23 (1.00 1.50)
Esophagus	1.15 (0.34 2.33)	1.12 (0.15 2.74)	0.87 (0.11 2.03)
Stomach	1.45 (1.11 1.89)	1.30 (0.93 1.80)	1.00 (0.68 1.43)
Colon	1.66 (0.75 3.02)	2.39 (1.01 4.85)	
Lung	1.62 (1.09 2.28)	1.57 (0.93 2.40)	1.64 (1.06 2.37)
Bladder and urinary tract	2.83 (1.19 6.02)	4.30 (1.78 11.01)	5.55 (1.17 89.74)
Female breast	4.01 (2.64 6.09)	3.81 (2.42 5.98)	2.52 (0.78 6.22)
Uterus	0.93 (0.57 1.36)	0.75 (0.40 1.15)	0.99 (0.34 1.86)
Rectum	1.94 (0.96 3.39)	1.98 (0.89 3.69)	
Pancreas	3.01 (1.52 5.69)	2.19 (0.68 5.17)	
Liver	1.29 (0.62 2.21)	1.35 (0.64 2.31)	
Gallbladder	0.76 (0.08 1.69)	0.83 (0.09 1.87)	
Ovary	0.48 (0.00 1.47)	1.06 (0.00 3.45)	
Prostate	2.15 (0.91 4.28)	2.26 (0.89 4.74)	
Thyroid	3.23 (2.02 5.03)	3.56 (2.17 5.73)	
Multiple myeloma	3.53 (1.11 9.95)	3.51 (0.64 13.06)	
Other lymphatic tissue	0.77 (0.22 1.50)	0.99 (0.29 1.99)	

[a] 0 rad used instead of 0–9 rad (90% confidence interval).

tality). Regardless of ascertainment method, relative risk was significantly increased for all malignancies, leukemia, all malignancies except leukemia, and cancer of the bladder, urinary tract, and thyroid in Nagasaki. In addition, significantly increased relative risks based on all methods of ascertainment were found for cancer of the stomach, lung, female breast, and pancreas, and multiple myeloma. Generally, estimates of relative risk derived by different ascertainment methods were similar.

As previously reported (*7*, *9*, *16*), a significant dose-response relationship pattern was observed for leukemia and cancer of the stomach, colon, liver, lung, breast, thyroid, prostate, and urinary tract, and multiple myeloma, as well as for all cancer sites (Fig. 3).

Estimates of absolute risk (excess cases per 10^6 person-year-rad (PYR)) were calculated under the assumption that the risk increases linearly with dose. The estimates based on three different ascertainment sources (all, confirmed, mortality) are shown in Table V. While relative risk estimates showed little differences by source of ascertainment, three estimates of absolute risk varied markedly. For all cancer sites, the absolute risk estimated from all sources was from two to five times higher than the risk estimated from mortality data only. Among various cancer sites, breast cancer showed the largest increase in absolute risk based on all methods over that based on mortality, followed by cancer of the stomach, lung, and uterus. Thus, absolute risk based on mortality data may underestimate the true risks for certain types of cancer. This may occur when cancer incidence is significantly higher than mortality. Such cancer may include relatively low lethal malignancies (such as breast cancer) and those with high incidence (*e.g.*, stomach and lung cancer).

Chronological changes of cancer risk in A-bomb survivors are of special interest for determining how long it takes before clinically evident cancer appears after radiation and

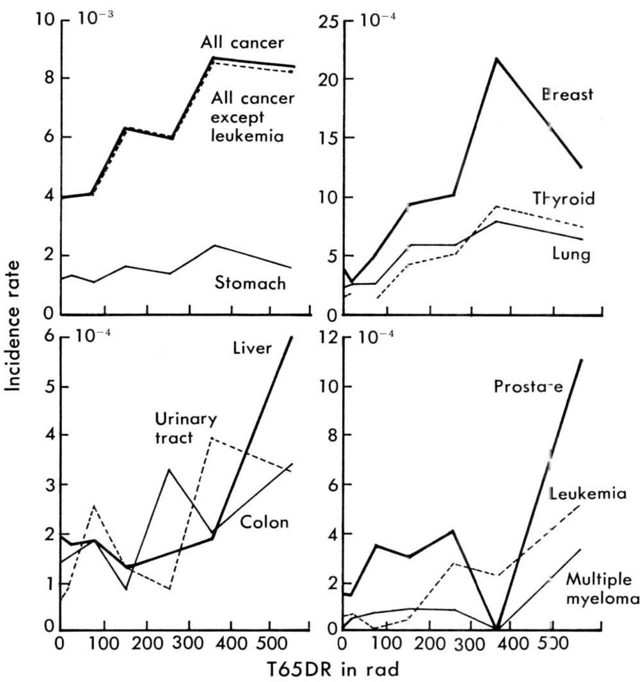

FIG. 3. Nagasaki Tumor Registry. Age-adjusted average annual incidence rate by dose for selected cancer sites, all methods of ascertainment, 1959–78.

TABLE V. Excess Cases per 10^6 PYR for All and Selected Cancer by Method of Ascertainment: Nagasaki, 1959–78

Site	Source		
	All sources	Confirmed	Mortality
All sites[a]	10.31 (8.27 12.35)	7.43 (5.70 9.17)	2.08 (0.60 3.55)
Leukemia	0.66 (0.41 0.92)	0.66 (0.41 0.92)	0.65 (0.41 0.90)
All except leukemia[a]	9.64 (7.62 11.67)	6.77 (5.05 8.48)	1.42 (−0.03 2.87)
Esophagus	−0.07 (−0.38 0.23)	−0.04 (−0.28 0.20)	−0.07 (−0.34 0.19)
Stomach	1.49 (0.38 2.59)	0.65 (−0.24 1.54)	0.23 (−0.60 1.06)
Colon	0.41 (0.04 0.77)	0.38 (0.08 0.69)	0.16 (−0.09 0.40)
Lung	0.87 (0.27 1.48)	0.65 (0.16 1.14)	0.55 (0.01 1.09)
Bladder and urinary tract	0.53 (0.22 0.84)	0.60 (0.32 0.88)	0.20 (0.01 0.40)
Female breast	3.30 (2.45 4.16)	2.57 (1.78 3.36)	0.31 (−0.12 0.73)
Uterus	0.09 (−1.01 1.18)	−0.45 (−1.45 0.56)	−0.24 (−0.81 0.33)
Rectum	0.34 (−0.03 0.71)	0.20 (−0.14 0.55)	
Pancreas	0.32 (−0.01 0.66)	0.03 (−0.22 0.28)	
Liver	0.45 (0.04 0.86)	0.49 (0.09 0.89)	
Gallbladder	−0.11 (−0.43 0.21)	−0.06 (−0.35 0.24)	
Salivary	−0.06 (−0.19 0.07)	−0.06 (−0.19 0.07)	
Ovary	−0.18 (−0.58 0.21)	−0.14 (−0.52 0.23)	
Thyroid	1.32 (0.88 1.76)	1.31 (0.90 1.72)	
Multiple myeloma	0.38 (0.17 0.60)	0.19 (0.03 0.34)	
Other lymphatic tissue	0.00 (−0.33 0.33)	0.11 (−0.19 0.40)	

[a] 0 rad used instead of 0–9 rad (90% confidence interval).

TABLE VI. Excess Incidence/10^6 PYR and 90% Confidence Limits by Period for Selected Sites of Cancer, Nagasaki, 1959–78

Period	Leukemia	All cancer except leukemia	Stomach
1959–62	2.29 (1.71 2.87)	7.97 (4.60 11.33)	1.83 (−0.04 3.71)
63–66	0.41 (−0.02 0.85)	6.10 (1.85 10.36)	1.26 (−1.12 3.63)
67–70	0.47 (−0.24 1.18)	7.24 (2.72 11.76)	0.42 (−2.29 3.14)
71–74	−0.08 (−0.37 0.22)	9.26 (4.11 14.41)	0.94 (−1.59 3.46)
75–78	−0.37 (−1.10 0.35)	19.65 (14.23 25.08)	2.91 (0.02 5.80)
Period	**Lung**	**Breast**	**Thyroid**
1959–62	1.46 (0.68 2.25)	−0.41 (−1.81 1.00)	2.34 (1.49 3.19)
63–66	0.54 (−0.64 1.72)	0.99 (−0.44 2.43)	1.11 (−0.10 2.32)
67–70	0.82 (−0.66 2.29)	8.62 (6.66 10.58)	0.71 (−0.19 1.61)
71–74	0.77 (−0.85 2.39)	1.95 (−0.27 4.18)	1.33 (0.37 2.30)
75–78	0.79 (−0.87 2.45)	5.86 (3.35 8.38)	1.56 (0.65 2.47)

(90% confidence interval).

how long carcinogenic effects of radiation persist. Table VI presents chronological change in absolute risk of leukemia and several other cancer sites. The excess incidence of leukemia decreased with time and reached zero by 1971, however, the excess risk for malignancies other than leukemia generally increased with time. Various reasons can be considered for the different latency periods for different tumors. For example, for malignancies such as lung and stomach cancer, radiation may play a relatively small role as compared with other initiating and promoting factors (*e.g.*, cigarette smoking, diet, and occupation). Host susceptibility such as age and endocrine factors may also be a significant factor in determining the time of clinical onset of some tumors (*e.g.*, breast and thyroid cancer).

The long-term follow-up of A-bomb survivors offers a unique opportunity for study of the latency period of cancer because of the well-defined time of single exposure. In determining the onset of cancer, incidence data provide a distinct advantage over mortality data. When using mortality data, one must assume that the case fatality or survival rate for a given type of tumor does not differ over calendar time and among different subgroups of interest (*e.g.*, age, sex, *etc.*). Such assumptions are not always justifiable.

Presentation of detailed incidence findings for specific types of cancer is beyond the scope of this paper and are discussed elsewhere in this monograph. However, it seems clear from what is already presented that incidence monitoring must be part of the continuing surveillance of health effects of A-bomb radiation exposure. Incidence data are needed 1) to assess the risk of developing relatively low lethal tumors such as cancer of the breast, thyroid, corpus uteri, *etc.*, 2) to improve diagnostic accuracy for both nonfatal (such as those mentioned above) and fatal (*e.g.*, pancreatic) cancer, and 3) to assess secular changes in carcinogenic effects of radiation. Tissue registry data should provide a unique opportunity for studying histological presentations of radiation-induced tumors, although these data have not been fully utilized. Reasons for difficulty in using tissue registry data include the possible selectivity of cases with histological diagnosis and the lack of clinical and other medical information needed for determining primary sites. The linkage of tumor and tissue registries should help resolve some of the problems.

REFERENCES

1. American Cancer Society. Manual of Tumor Nomenclature and Coding (1968). American Cancer Society, Inc., New York.
2. Belsky, J. L., Takeichi, N., Yamamoto, T., Cihak, R. W., Hirose, F., Ezaki, H., Inoue, S., and Blot, W. J. Salivary gland neoplasms following atomic radiation: Additional cases and reanalysis of combined data in a fixed population, 1957–1970. *Cancer*, **35**, 555–559 (1975).
3. Freedman, L. A., Fukushima, K., and Seigel, D. G. ABCC-JNIH Adult Health Study, Report 4, 1960–62 cycle examination, Hiroshima and Nagasaki. ABCC Tech. Rep. 20-63 (1963).
4. Hanai, A., Kitamura, H., Fukuma, S., and Fujimoto, I. (ed.) Cancer incidence in Japan 1975–1979 (1984). The Osaka Cancer Registry, Osaka.
5. Harada, T., Ide, M., Ishida, M., and Troup, G. M. Malignant Neoplasms, Tumor Registry Data. Hiroshima and Nagasaki 1957–59. Report of the Research Committee on Tumor Statistics, Hiroshima and Nagasaki City Medical Association. ABCC Tech. Rep. 23-63 (1963).
6. Harada, T. and Ishida, M. Neoplasms among A-bomb survivors in Hiroshima; First Report of the Research Committee on Tumor Statistics, Hiroshima City Medical Association, Hiroshima, Japan. *J. Natl. Cancer Inst.*, **25**, 1253–1264 (1960).
7. Ichimaru, M., Ishimaru, T., and Belsky, J. L. Incidence of leukemia in atomic bomb survivors belonging to a fixed cohort in Hiroshima and Nagasaki, 1950–71: Radiation dose, years after exposure, age at exposure, and type of leukemia. *J. Radiat. Res.*, **19**, 262–282 (1978).
8. Ishida, M. Statistical Aspect of Tumor Registries in Hiroshima and Nagasaki. *Bull. Int. Stat. Inst.*, **38**, 233–234 (1961).
9. Kato, H. and Schull, W. J. Studies of the mortality of A-bomb survivors. Report 7. Mortality 1950–1978: Part I. Cancer mortality. *Radiat. Res.*, **90**, 395–432 (1982).
10. Kerr, G. D. and Soloman, D. L. The epicenter of the Nagasaki weapon: A reanalysis of available data with recommended values. Oak Ridge National Laboratory, Oak Ridge, TN, 1976.
11. Maclennan, R., Muir, C. S., Steinitz, R., and Winkler, A. (ed.) Cancer Registration and Its Techniques. International Agency for Research on Cancer (IARC) Scientific Publication No. 21 (1978).
12. Matsuura, H., Yamamoto, T., Sekine, I., Ichi, Y., and Otake, M. Pathological and epidemiological study of gastric cancer in atomic bomb survivors, Hiroshima and Nagasaki, 1955–57. *Radiat. Res.*, **25**, 111–129 (1984).
13. McGregor, D. H., Land, C. E., Choi, K., Tokuoka, S., Lin, P. I., Wakabayashi, T., and Beebe, G. W. Breast cancer incidence among atomic bomb survivors, Hiroshima and Nagasaki, 1950–69. *J. Natl. Cancer Inst.*, **59**, 799–811 (1977).
14. Nakatsuka, H. and Ezaki, H. Colorectal cancer among atomic bomb survivors, this volume, pp. 157–167.
15. Schull, W. J. and Masaki, K. Dosimetry studies information. Documents prepared for RERF seventh meeting of the scientific councillors, 17–19 March 1980.
16. Tokunaga, M., Norman, J. E., Jr., Asano, M., Tokuoka, S., Ezaki, H., Nishimori, I., and Tsuji, Y. Malignant breast tumors among atomic bomb survivors, Hiroshima and Nagasaki, 1950–74. *J. Natl. Cancer Inst.*, **62**, 1347–1359 (1979).
17. Wakabayashi, T., Kato, H., Ikeda, T., and Schull, W. J. Studies of the mortality of A-bomb survivors, Report 7. Part III. Increase of cancer in 1959–1978, based on the Tumor Registry, Nagasaki. *Radiat. Res.*, **93**, 112–146 (1983).
18. Wanebo, C. K., Johnson, K. G., Sato, K., and Thorslund, T. W. Breast cancer after ex-

posure to the atomic bombings of Hiroshima and Nagasaki. *N. Engl. J. Med.*, **279**, 667–671 (1968).

19. Wanebo, C. K., Johnson, K. G., Sato, K., and Thorslund, T. W. Lung cancer following atomic radiation. *Am. Rev. Respir. Dis.*, **88**, 778–787 (1968).
20. World Health Organization. International Classification of Diseases for Oncology (1976). WHO, Geneva.
21. World Health Organization. Manual of the International Statistical Classification of Diseases. Injuries and Causes of Death (1977). WHO, Geneva.
22. Wood, J. W., Tamagaki, H., Neriishi, S., Sato, T., Sheldon, W. F., Archer, P. G., Hamilton, H. B., and Johnson, K. G. Thyroid carcinoma in atomic bomb survivors, Hiroshima and Nagasaki. *Am. J. Epidemiol.*, **89**, 4–14 (1969).
23. Yamamoto, T., Nishimori, I., Tahara, E., and Sekine, I. Malignant tumors in atomic bomb survivors with special reference to the pathology of stomach and lung cancer, this volume, pp. 145–156.

GANN Monograph on Cancer Research 32, 1986

THE CANCER REGISTRY IN NAGASAKI CITY, WITH ATOMIC BOMB SURVIVOR DATA, 1973–1977

Takayoshi IKEDA, Ichiro HAYASHI, Takeshi MATSUO, Hiroshi MAEDA, and Isao SHIMOKAWA

*First Department of Pathology, Nagasaki University School of Medicine**

The tumor registry program in Nagasaki City was conceived as a contribution to knowledge concerning possible radiation induced carcinogenesis among a human population and a tumor registry was established in 1957 and a tissue registry in 1974.

According to the chronological changes in adjusted incidence rates for Nagasaki City, an increasing trend was shown in males for cancer of the colon, rectum, lung, urinary bladder, and for all sites combined, and, in females for cancer of the colon, pancreas, and breast. No decreasing trend was observed for any site in males, while a decreasing trend was indicated in females for cancer of the uterus.

In comparison with age-adjusted incidence rates for all cancer sites combined in other prefectures and cities in 1979, the rates in Nagasaki City are high for both males and females. Sites with a tendency for high rates, in Nagasaki City, are, for males, stomach, colon, rectum, liver, and lymphoid tissue, and for females, colon, rectum, liver, gallbladder, lung, breast, and lymphoid tissue.

From these data, it is necessary to ascertain whether or not the incidence of malignant tumors is higher among atomic bomb (A-bomb) survivors than in nonexposed persons. According to the Nagasaki City tumor and tissue registry data for 1973–77, the crude incidence rate and relative risk for several cancers were higher in A-bomb survivors and well correlated with the radiation dose. However, the adjusted relative risk showed a higher trend only for thyroid cancer in females and in double cancers for both sexes. Histopathological difference between cancer tissue of A-bomb survivors and nonexposed persons was not detected.

In general, it is premature to determine the qualitative and quantitative differences of malignancy between A-bomb survivors and nonexposed persons, although an increase in cancer incidence and mortality is a recognized late effect of exposure to A-bomb radiation in Hiroshima and Nagasaki.

The purpose of a population based cancer registry is to determine the magnitude of the effect of tumors, especially malignant tumors, on the community so as to help control the malignancy. Registration is an effective means of epidemiological research to inquire into the cause of malignant tumors, and provides data concerning geopathological differences in carcinogenesis in establishing an epidemiological hypothesis.

The specific purpose of the Nagasaki City Tumor Registry is to ascertain whether or

* Sakamoto-machi 12-4, Nagasaki 852, Japan (池田高良, 林　一郎, 松尾　武, 前田　公, 下川　功).

not the incidence of malignant tumors is higher among atomic bomb (A-bomb) survivors than in nonexposed populations.

The Nagasaki City Tumor Statistics Committee was established in Nagasaki City in 1957 as a special committee of the Nagasaki City Medical Association, and tumor registration has been conducted in cooperation with the Radiation Effects Research Foundation (RERF, formerly the Atomic Bomb Casualty Commission) for 27 years. In September 1974, the Nagasaki Neoplasm Tissue Registry Commission was established with a research grant from the U.S. National Cancer Institute, and tissue registration has been carried out jointly.

To improve the accuracy of tumor registration, the use of the International Classification of Diseases (ICD-O) code was recommended in 1976 and a tendency has developed to use this code throughout the world. Histological type has to be considered in epidemiological and clinical studies because it is often related to etiology and prognosis and the ICD-O code makes histological typing of all malignant tumors possible. However, because ICD-O is a classification of histological type, participation of at least one pathologist is necessary in its use. For example, terminology and diagnostic criteria often differ among schools and ICD evaluation by pathologists is necessary. In Nagasaki City, the tissue registry was established in addition to the tumor registry, and these two committees are cooperating.

Population Based Cancer Registry Data

Population based cancer registration is conducted in 13 prefectures and 2 cities in Japan (*2*, *8*, *9*). One of the main purposes of a population based cancer registration is

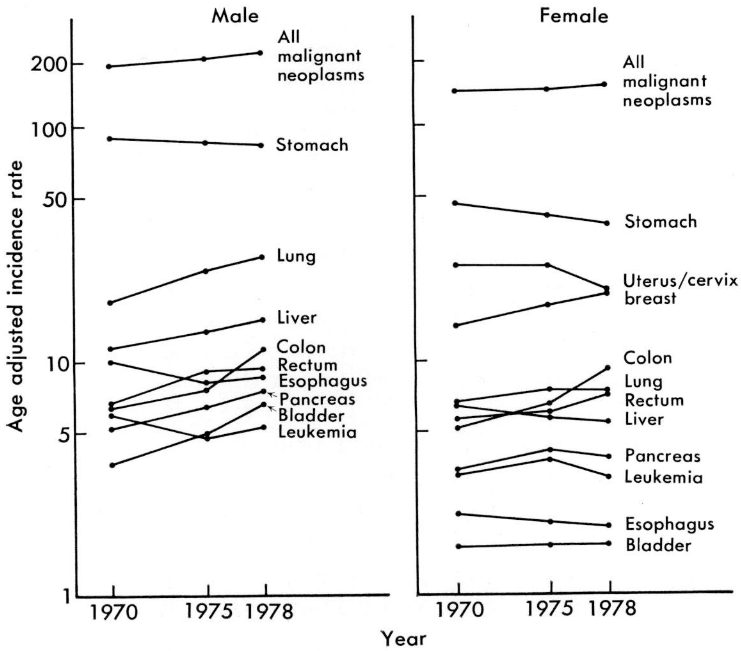

FIG. 1. Chronological changes in estimated incidence rate, Japan 1970, 1975, and 1978.

to determine incidence rates and observe chronological changes. Cancer registration establishes the direction of cancer countermeasures and contributes to epidemiological research on cancer. In Japan, few registry offices possess long period incidence data with moderate accuracy. In these 13 prefectures and 2 cities, both incidence and mortality rates show a slight but gradual rising tendency in recent years as shown in Fig. 1 (*2*). According to the chronological changes in age-adjusted incidence rates for main cancer sites in Nagasaki, an increasing trend is shown in males for the colon, rectum, lung, urinary bladder, and all sites combined, and an increasing trend in females for the colon, pancreas, and breast. No decreasing trend is observed for any site in males, while a decreasing trend is indicated in females for cancer of the uterus. A peculiar finding in Nagasaki is no decreasing trend for stomach cancer in males compared with other regions.

The proportion of cases based only on death certificates is used as an index of the

TABLE I. Chronological Changes of the Rate of Cases Based on the Death Certificate in Four Regions of Japan (% of Cases with Malignancy)

Region	Year					
	1975	1976	1977	1978	1979	1980
A	23.9	21.5	21.8	18.3	16.5	14.1
B	29.2	26.5	29.0	28.5	26.0	26.6
C	22.9	19.6	21.5	15.3	14.1	14.5
D[a]	10.4	8.2	8.0	3.0	9.0	6.1

[a] Nagasaki City.

TABLE II. Chronological Changes of the Rate of Cases Based on Histological Diagnosis in Four Regions of Japan (% of All Malignancies)

Region	Year					
	1975	1976	1977	1978	1979	1980
A	58.0	59.6	59.1	64.2	64.1	69.1
B	38.5	43.1	43.0	51.2	56.7	58.4
C	69.4	69.4	63.6	69.3	69.4	72.4
D[a]	67.1	67.1	72.9	76.2	74.3	77.0

[a] Nagasaki City.

TABLE III. Incidence and Mortality Rates for All Sites by Sex in Six Regions of Japan, 1979

Region	Male		Female	
	Incidence	Mortality	Incidence	Mortality
A	218.7	148.8	142.9	85.2
E	218.5	156.6	140.1	90.2*
F	183.0	145.5	122.8**	84.5
B	220.2	160.5*	148.0	91.6*
C	310.8*	153.7	219.5*	80.2
D	266.2*	177.2*	174.2*	100.6*
Mean	207.1	150.4	141.2	86.7
S.D.	11.7	3.7	8.2	1.7

* mean+2 S.D.
** mean−2 S.D.

TABLE IV. Adjusted Incidence Rates by Sex and Site[a] in Four Regions of Japan, 1979

ICD	Site	Male				Female			
		A	B	C	D[b]	A	B	C	D[b]
140–209	All malignant neoplasms	218.7	220.2	310.8	266.2	142.9	148.0	219.5	174.2
150	Esophagus	13.6	7.9	11.6	9.2	3.7	1.9	1.9	1.1
151	Stomach	82.0	73.9	98.9	88.9	35.9	37.8	43.6	37.1
153	Colon	8.0	9.8	14.0	13.4	8.9	7.2	10.7	10.6
154	Rectum	9.4	9.4	16.3	10.9	7.2	5.4	9.2	10.0
155	Liver	11.6	25.9	20.9	27.1	4.3	7.0	8.7	11.1
156	Gallbladder, bile duct	6.6	3.7	3.5	7.4	5.6	3.8	3.2	7.3
157	Pancreas	10.6	7.1	8.8	5.4	5.4	4.8	4.3	3.1
161	Larynx	1.7	4.0	7.3	3.1	0.2	0.5	0.7	0.3
162	Lung	30.3	32.8	43.0	30.2	8.3	10.5	12.2	10.7
174, 175	Breast	0.2	0.2	0.0	0.4	21.0	17.3	36.2	22.7
179–182 233.1	Uterus Cervix *in situ* }	—	—	—	—	15.9	27.1	40.3	27.2
183.0	Ovary	—	—	—	—	4.2	3.7	6.3	6.1
185	Prostate	5.7	4.7	9.1	9.4	—	—	—	—
188	Bladder	6.5	6.0	12.1	15.4	1.6	1.8	3.1	2.2
200–203	Lymphatic except leukemia	6.6	5.1	11.4	9.3	4.0	3.6	4.9	6.6
204–208	Leukemia	6.1	4.7	8.2	5.5	3.8	3.2	3.4	0.0
233.1	Cervix *in situ*	—	—	—	—	2.4	4.3	5.9	2.2

[a] Adjusted to world population.
[b] Nagasaki City.

TABLE V. Adjusted Mortality Rates by Sex and Site[a] in Four Regions of Japan, 1979

ICD	Site	Male				Female			
		A	B	C	D[b]	A	B	C	D[b]
140–209	All malignant neoplasms	148.8	160.5	153.7	177.2	85.2	91.6	80.2	100.6
150	Esophagus	10.6	6.4	4.5	4.5	2.5	1.4	1.3	0.0
151	Stomach	48.1	52.5	48.1	43.8	24.3	26.9	24.6	22.6
153	Colon	5.4	6.2	4.9	6.1	4.2	4.7	2.9	4.5
154	Rectum	6.9	6.8	4.5	7.3	5.2	3.6	3.3	5.1
155	Liver	10.4	22.3	21.9	30.1	4.4	6.5	6.4	10.5
156	Gallbladder, bile duct	4.9	3.2	3.3	7.0	5.3	2.9	2.7	6.1
157	Pancreas	9.0	6.2	5.6	6.8	4.3	4.5	3.0	3.4
161	Larynx	1.3	1.6	1.4	0.5	0.4	0.2	0.3	0.0
162	Lung	22.2	28.8	29.1	32.9	7.4	8.8	6.3	9.9
174, 175	Breast	0.1	0.1	0.6	0.0	5.0	5.2	4.9	7.4
179–182 233.1	Uterus Cervix *in situ* }	—	—	—	—	5.3	9.6	8.8	8.9
183.0	Ovary	—	—	—	—	1.9	2.6	3.5	2.9
185	Prostate	2.5	2.3	2.0	2.5	—	—	—	—
188	Bladder	2.5	2.5	2.9	3.2	1.1	0.9	0.7	1.7
200–203	Lymphatic except leukemia	5.2	4.2	5.9	9.9	2.1	2.5	0.9	6.1
204–208	Leukemia	5.2	3.8	5.5	5.7	3.6	2.7	2.5	1.5
233.1	Cervix *in situ*	—	—	—	—	0.0	0.0	0.0	0.0

[a] Adjusted to world population.
[b] Nagasaki City.

accuracy of registration, especially the accuracy of reporting. The reliability of incidence rates is higher when the proportion based only on death certificates is lower. Another index of registration accuracy is the rate of histological diagnosis. The higher the rate of histological diagnosis, the higher becomes the accuracy of the registration. In Nagasaki City, both the proportion of cases based only on death certificates (less than 10%) and the histological diagnosis rate (more than 70%) recently show excellent values (Tables I and II). In comparison with the adjusted incidence rates for all sites among the prefectures and cities in 1979 that are conducting population based cancer registries, the rate is remarkably high in both males and females of Nagasaki City (Table III). The sites showing an increasing tendency of rate in males of Nagasaki City are the stomach, colon, rectum, liver, and lymphoid tissues, and in females, the colon, rectum, liver, gallbladder, lung, breast, and lymphoid tissues (Table IV). Adjusted mortality rates by site (Table V) show a similar trend to adjusted incidence rates (*2*).

Nagasaki City A-bomb Survivor Data

In general, a higher trend of cancer incidence rates in a certain region is reflected by geographically specific phenomena or by the influence of known or unknown factors, such as air pollution, radiation, *etc.* Geographically, Nagasaki City is located in southwestern Japan by the sea, and a possible factor influencing cancer incidence may be the existence of a particular group (*i.e.*, A-bomb survivors) in the population. The former factor has not been investigated so far, but it has been noted that the frequency of malignant lymphoma, especially the T-cell type, and of liver cancer are higher in Nagasaki Prefecture and in the southwestern part of Japan than in other areas. The pathogenesis of these malignant tumors has been postulated as involvement of viruses, retrovirus or hepatitis B virus. The latter factors have been studied extensively. According to a report on a fixed population of the RERF Life Span Study (LSS) using the tumor registry data in Nagasaki City during the period 1959–78, a higher trend of cancer incidence was noted in several sites, such as leukemia, and cancer of the lung, breast, stomach, and thyroid gland (*13*). Furthermore, a suggestively higher trend in incidence was observed in cancer of the colon and urinary tract, and in multiple myeloma. In this study, the dose estimates were based on the RERF revised T65 dose system.

As previously described, the rate of histological diagnosis in Nagasaki City was more than 70% for all sites combined in recent years and it may be enough to evaluate the histological types of malignancy in the population by exposure status. For this reason, the authors have investigated, in addition to the population based incidence rates, the pathohistological type of malignancy in several organs by exposure status of survivors in Nagasaki City for five years (1973–77). An exposed person was defined as one who was exposed to the A-bomb directly within 10,000 m from ground zero or who entered the city within two weeks after the bombing. Data of exposure status was prepared by the Data Center of the A-Bomb Disaster, Nagasaki University School of Medicine. In 1975, the middle year of the investigation period, A-bomb survivors in Nagasaki City numbered about 82,000 (18%) among the population of about 450,000 and most A-bomb survivors were already 30 or more years old. Thus, among the population aged 30 years or more, 37.8% were A-bomb survivors (Table VI). This means A-bomb survivors were reaching or had already reached the so-called "cancer age."

The other problem noted was the age distribution of A-bomb survivors, which was

Early entry		0.58	1.06	1.31	0.45	1.81	0.87	1.00
Total	2.37	1.09	0.72	0.99	0.59	1.10	2.06	0.86

TABLE VI. Population of Nagasaki City, 1975

2. *Lung cancer (3)*

There were 435 cases (170 exposed and 265 nonexposed) of lung cancer registered (Table X). Crude incidence rate was higher in A-bomb survivors for both sexes, but no significant difference in the age-adjusted rate was noted compared with nonexposed persons. Relative risk was slightly higher in the exposed, especially for early entrants of both sexes, although age-adjusted relative risk was not significant. The incidence rate by age group was not significant between the exposed and nonexposed. By histological type, adenocarcinoma was the most frequent in both sexes and in both the exposed and nonexposed, followed by squamous cell carcinoma, large cell carcinoma including mucin-like contents, and small cell carcinoma. In A-bomb survivors, adenocarcinoma was more frequent in males and less frequent in females compared with the nonexposed.

TABLE X. Incidence Rates, Relative Risk, and Age-adjusted Relative Risk (*vs.* nonexposed) for Lung Cancer in Cases Aged 30 Years or More, Nagasaki City, 1973–77

Sex	Rate and risk	Exposure (distance from ground zero)					Nonexposed
		<2,000 m	2,000–9,999 m	<9,999 m	Early entry	Total	
Male	Crude incidence rate[a]	66.5	63.7	64.1	104.1	71.6	57.1
	Relative risk	1.17	1.12	1.12	1.83	1.26	1.00
	Age-adjusted relative risk			0.77		0.80	1.00
Female	Crude incidence rate[a]	24.6	25.1	25.1	31.5	26.0	19.3
	Relative risk	1.27	1.30	1.30	1.63	1.35	1.00
	Age-adjusted relative risk			0.90		0.93	1.00

[a] Incidence rate per 100,000.

3. *Thyroid cancer (5)*

There were 89 cases (38 exposed and 51 nonexposed) of thyroid cancer registered (Table XI). The incidence rate tended to be higher in A-bomb survivors, especially in females, than in the nonexposed. Compared with the nonexposed, the relative risk of incidence was increased in the proximally and distally exposed, but not for early entrants. Among 83 cases examined histologically, papillary adenocarcinoma was predominant, and was more prevalent in the exposed than in the nonexposed. Age distribution of the exposed was similar to the nonexposed.

TABLE XI. Incidence Rates and Relative Risk (*vs.* nonexposed) for Thyroid Cancer in Cases Aged 30 Years or More by Exposure Status and Sex, Nagasaki City, 1973–77

Sex	Rate and risk	Exposure (distance from ground zero)			Nonexposed
		<2,000 m	2,000–9,999 m	Early entry	
Male	Crude incidence rate[a]	5.5	4.7	3.5	2.9
	Relative risk	1.90	1.60	1.19	1.00
Female	Crude incidence rate[a]	24.6	12.0	9.5	8.9
	Relative risk	2.75	1.34	1.06	1.00

[a] Incidence rate per 100,000.

4. *Colon cancer (11)*

There were 223 cases (84 exposed and 139 nonexposed) of colon cancer registered.

The incidence in A-bomb survivors was not significantly different compared with the nonexposed. By site, cancer of the sigmoid colon was more frequent in males than in females, particularly in the older age groups, but no difference was noted by exposure status. The relative risk was 0.96 in males and 1.33 in females, although no significant difference was noted in age-adjusted relative risk. Histologically about 90% of the cases were of relatively differentiated adenocarcinoma, and showed no difference by age, sex, or exposure status.

5. *Multiple primary malignancies* (7)

There were 94 cases (43 exposed and 51 nonexposed) of multiple primary malignancies registered as the second or third malignancy during 1973–77 (Tables XII and XIII). The rate of histological diagnosis by site was difficult to determine, so the rate for all sites combined was used in this study. The average age at the time of the first and second malignancies was younger in females than in males, and by exposure status, the age at the first and second malignancies was older in male and younger in female A-bomb survivors than in the nonexposed. As far as only double cancers are concerned, the average interval between the occurrence of the first and second malignancies was 0.7 years for exposed males and 3.0 years for exposed females, whereas it was 1.7 years for nonexposed males and 2.7 years for nonexposed females. Thus, more than half of the cases had developed the second tumor within a one year period. Stomach cancer was the most frequent (50%) followed by breast cancer (15%). The incidence rate and relative risk were higher in both sexes of the exposed compared with the nonexposed, and the age adjusted relative risk was 1.27 in males and 1.13 in females.

In summary of the data of A-bomb survivors for 1973–77 (Table XIV), several trends may be suggested or demonstrated as follows: 1) Crude incidence rates and

TABLE XII. Average Age at the Time of First, Second, and Third Malignant Tumor by Exposure Status and Sex, Nagasaki City, 1973–77

Malignant Tumor	Exposed		Nonexposed	
	Male	Female	Male	Female
First	67.2	55.3	62.8	60.0
Second	68.7	58.6	64.6	63.4
Third	64.0	33.0	67.3	66.7

TABLE XIII. Incidence Rates and Relative Risk of Multiple Primary Malignant Tumors in Cases Aged 30 Years or More by Exposure Status and Sex, Nagasaki City, 1973–77

Sex	Rate and risk	Exposure (distance from ground zero)			Nonexposed	Total
		<9,999 m	Early entry	Total		
Male	Crude incidence rate[a]	16.76	14.52	16.35	10.20	12.09
	Relative risk	1.64	1.42	1.60	1.00	1.19
	Age-adjusted relative risk	—	—	1.27	1.00	—
Female	Crude incidence rate[a]	13.16	20.19	14.19	9.53	11.36
	Relative risk	1.38	2.17	1.49	1.00	1.19
	Age-adjusted relative risk	—	—	1.13	1.00	—

[a] Incidence rate per 100,000.

TABLE XIV. Crude Incidence Rates and Relative Risk by Site and Exposure Status, Cases Aged 30 Years or More, Nagasaki City, 1973–77

Sex	Site	Incidence			Relative risk	
		Exposed	Nonexposed	X	Not adjusted	Adjusted[a]
Male	Stomach	196.6	171.7	NS	1.72	0.89
	Lung	71.6	57.1	NS	1.26	0.80
	Thyroid	4.6	2.9	NS	1.59	
	Colon	22.1	23.1	NS	0.96	0.68
	Double Cancer	11.7	7.3	NS	1.60	1.27
Female	Stomach	94.7	83.9	S	1.72	0.87
	Lung	26.0	19.3	NS	1.35	0.93
	Thyroid	13.4	8.9	NS	1.51	1.29
	Colon	21.6	16.2	NS	1.33	1.04
	Double Cancer	10.8	7.3	NS	1.48	1.13

X, Mantel-Haenszel test.
[a] Calculated by Miettinen method.
S, Significant *vs.* nonexposed (<2,000 m).
NS, Not significant *vs.* nonexposed.

relative risk were higher in A-bomb survivors than those in the nonexposed, but the age-adjusted relative risk was not significantly different between them in most malignant tumors investigated. This does not mean that exposure to radiation is not related to cancer induction during the period investigated. 2) The relative risk of these malignancies was well correlated with the radiation dose (distance from ground zero), and the risk for the early entrants was higher in most sites than the survivors exposed at 2,000 m or more. 3) For stomach cancer the relative risk was higher in younger people exposed to radiation at less than 2,000 m from ground zero. Thus, those exposed to radiation at a younger age might be susceptible to malignancies, although malignancies of other sites were not assessable because of the small number of subjects in each age group examined. 4) In A-bomb survivors, the age adjusted relative risk was higher in females for lung, colon, and thyroid cancer and was higher in males for multiple cancer. 5) For double cancer, the age at the first tumor was higher in exposed males than in nonexposed males, while it was lower in exposed females than in nonexposed females. A similar trend was observed for the second malignancy. The trend of lower age in exposed females might be reflected by the earlier occurrence of inherent cancer in younger females such as cancer of the breast and uterine cervix, but the reason for early or late occurrence of the first and second tumors in females or males of the exposed was not elucidated in this study.

At present, an increase in cancer incidence and mortality is an indisputable late effect of exposure to A-bomb radiation in Hiroshima and Nagasaki. According to a cohort study by RERF, it is demonstrated that mortality from malignant tumors among A-bomb survivors is higher in Hiroshima than in Nagasaki. Furthermore, organs involved in elevated risk of cancer are more numerous in Hiroshima than in Nagasaki (*6*). These data may indicate that biological effect of exposure to neutrons is generally greater than gamma radiation (*1*), but the new dosimetry indicates that this interpretation is incorrect.

The histological type of cancer has been suggested to differ in incidence by cause such as environmental factors and sex. The difference in histology between radiation induced cancer and spontaneous cancer is still equivocal at present. For breast cancer, the histological type is not different between the exposed and nonexposed, although the incidence is higher in A-bomb survivors (*12*). A similar situation is observed in stomach cancer where poorly differentiated adenocarcinoma is more frequent in A-bomb survivors than in the nonexposed (*10*). Adenocarcinoma of the lung is more frequent especially in exposed males than in the others (*3*). However, these data are not adequate to be decisive.

Thus, in general, it is premature to determine the qualitative differences of malignancy between A-bomb survivors and the nonexposed. Further investigation and accumulation of data are required.

CONCLUSION

A population based cancer registration is a useful means for detection of the cause or related factors of carcinogenesis. In fact, a cohort study or population based cancer registration has contributed to clarifying a higher trend of malignant lymphoma and liver cancer, and also of malignancy in A-bomb survivors in Nagasaki City. At present, A-bomb survivors are reaching or have reached those ages at which the incidence of cancer is elevated. Under these circumstances, it is necessary to investigate continuously the chronological changes of cancer incidence and the trend of incidence by histological type of malignancy in every organ to evaluate radiation induced carcinogenesis.

Acknowledgments

The authors express their sincere appreciation to all members of the Nagasaki Tumor Registry Committee of the Nagasaki City Medical Association for allowing the use of the registry data on tumors, and to all members of the Department of Epidemiology and Statistics, RERF for providing the cancer registry data. The authors also express their gratitude to Mrs. Mariko Mine, the Data Center for A-Bomb Disaster, Nagasaki University School of Medicine, for providing the data of exposure status.

REFERENCES

1. Fujita, S., Shimizu, Y., Yoshimoto, K., Yoshimoto, Y., and Kato, H. RBE of neutron in cancer mortality among atomic bomb survivors, Hiroshima and Nagasaki, 1950–1978. RERF Tech. Rep. 9-80, 1–19 (1983).
2. Fukuma, S. Studies on the Correlation between Environmental Factors and Treatment of Cancers in Cancer Registries. Progress Report Contract No. 56–2, Ministry of Health and Welfare (1983) (in Japanese).
3. Ide, M., Matsuo, T., Shimokawa, I., Mine, H., Maeda, H., and Ikeda, T. Epidemiology of Lung Cancer in Nagasaki—Especially in relation to radiation exposure. *Jpn. J. Cancer Clin.*, **30**, 334–339 (1984) (in Japanese).
4. Iwasaki, K., Kawamoto, K., Shimokawa, I., Matsuo, T., and Ikeda, T. Epidemiological Studies on Gastric Cancer in Nagasaki *Jpn. J. Cancer Clin.*, **30**, 1746–1754 (1984) (in Japanese).
5. Jubashi, T., Matsuo, T., Shimokawa, I., Wago, M., and Ikeda, T. Epidemiological Studies on Thyroid Cancer in Nagasaki City. *Jpn. J. Cancer Clin.*, **30**, 459–465 (1984) (in Japanese).
6. Kurihara, M., Munaka, M., Hayakawa, N., Yamamoto, H., Ueoka, H., and Ohtaki, M. Mortality Statistics among Atomic Bomb Survivors in Hiroshima Prefecture, 1968–1972. *J. Radiat. Res.*, **22**, 456–471 (1981)

7. Murase, K., Shimokawa, I., Hayashida, M., Matsuo, T., and Ideda, T. Epidemiological Studies on Multiple Primary Malignant Tumors in Nagasaki City. *Jpn. J. Cancer Clin.*, **30**, 871–879 (1984) (in Japanese).
8. Research Group for Population-based Cancer Registration in Japan. Cancer Incidence in Japan, 1975—Cancer Registry Statistics, *In* "Cancer Mortality and Morbidity Statistics" (GANN Monograph on Cancer Research No. 26), ed. M. Segi *et al.*, pp. 92–116 (1981). Japan Sci. Soc. Press, Tokyo.
9. Research Group for Population Based Cancer Registration in Japan. Prediction of the Future Incidence of Cancer in Japan. *Jpn. J. Clin. Oncol.*, **12**, 65–72 (1982).
10. Sekine, I., Nishimori, I., Matsuura, H., Yamamoto, T., and Ochi, Y. Pathological and epidemiological studies of gastric cancer in atomic bomb survivors (1950–1977, Hiroshima and Nagasaki). *Annu. Rep. Res. Assoc. Late Effect A-Bomb*, **23**, 105–112 (1982).
11. Shimokawa, I., Matsuo, T., Matsuo, S. and Ikeda, T. Epidemiological Studies of Colon Cancer in Nagasaki City, with special reference to radiation exposure. *Jpn. J. Cancer Clin.*, **30**, 1269–1273 (1984) (in Japanese).
12. Tokunaga, M., Norman, J. E., Jr., Asano, M., Tokuoka, S., Ezaki, H., Nishimori, I., and Tsuji, I. Malignant breast tumors among atomic bomb survivors, Hiroshima and Nagasaki, 1950–1974. *J. Natl. Cancer Inst.*, **62**, 1347–1359 (1979).
13. Wakabayashi, T., Kato, H., Ikeda, T., and Schull, W. J. Studies of the Mortality of A-Bomb Survivors, Report 7: Part III. Incidence of Cancer in 1959–1978, Based on the Tumor Registry, Nagasaki. *Radiat. Res.*, **93**, 112–146 (1983).

CANCER MORTALITY

Hiroo KATO

Department of Epidemiology and Statistics,
*Radiation Effects Research Foundation**

The Radiation Effects Research Foundation (RERF) and its predecessor, the Atomic Bomb Casualty Commission (ABCC), have conducted mortality surveillance on a fixed sample, the Life Span Study (LSS), of 82,000 atomic bomb (A-bomb) survivors and 27,000 nonexposed residents of Hiroshima and Nagasaki since 1950. The results of the most recent analysis of the LSS can be summarized as follows:

1. As a late effect of A-bomb radiation, mortality from malignant tumors increased among A-bomb survivors. Besides, the well-known increase of leukemia, cancer of the lung, breast, stomach, colon, and thyroid, and multiple myeloma also increased, but no increase in mortality from cancer of the rectum and uterus has yet been observed.

2. An increase in leukemia mortality among A-bomb survivors began to appear 2–3 years after exposure and reached a peak within 5–6 years. Thereafter, it decreased. For Hiroshima, however, the mortality rate is still slightly higher than the control level, even in the most recent period of observation from 1974–78. The pattern of appearance over time of radiation-induced cancer other than leukemia, however, differs from that of leukemia. In general, radiation-induced solid cancer begins to appear after the age is attained at which the cancer is normally prone to develop (so-called cancer age), and has continued to increase proportionately with the increase in mortality of the control group as it ages.

3. There are factors which modify the effect of radiation, such as age at the time of the bomb (ATB). Sensitivity to radiation, in terms of cancer induction, is higher for persons who were young ATB in general than for those who were older ATB.

4. The number of excess deaths from cancer among A-bomb survivors has been estimated. Results indicate that 50% of the leukemia deaths and 3.5% of the deaths due to all cancer except leukemia that have occurred in the LSS sample during the period 1950–78 are attributable to A-bomb radiation.

5. The relationship between radiation and other carcinogens such as tobacco has been investigated. There seems to be no interaction in a multiplicative way between radiation and smoking in lung cancer induction. Rather, the joint effect seems more consistent with an additive model.

The Atomic Bomb Casualty Commission (ABCC) and the Radiation Effects Research Foundation (RERF) have conducted mortality surveillance on a fixed sample (Life Span Study (LSS)) of 82,000 atomic bomb (A-bomb) survivors and 27,000 nonexposed residents of Hiroshima and Nagasaki since 1950 (*2*, *3*). The LSS was designed to identify and

* Hijiyama Park 5-2, Minami-ku, Hiroshima 732, Japan (加藤寛夫).

measure the possible late effects of acute radiation exposure from the A-bombs expressed through mortality overall or by specific disease categories. Its strength is that mortality ascertainment is essentially complete, regardless of a person's address in Japan, due to the periodic check of Koseki records of the LSS sample members. Its weakness is its reliance on the cause of death as stated on the death certificate. Some of the misclassification that can arise is compensated for by collateral use of autopsy information and data from the Hiroshima and Nagasaki Tissue and Tumor Registries (*34*).

Periodic analyses of the mortality experience of the LSS sample continue; the most recently published account spanned the years 1950–78 (*15*, *16*). The late effects of A-bomb radiation on mortality have been limited, so far, to an excess mortality from malignant neoplasms and not from other causes of death. No shortening of life-span due to causes other than malignant neoplasms was observed. Thus, the results obtained do not support the nonspecific acceleration of aging due to radiation.

With the ongoing accumulation of data, the most recent analysis addresses problems which previous publications were able to treat less well because of a small number of deaths (*16*). Issues such as the latent period for radiation-related malignancies and the effects of age at the time of the bomb (ATB) as well as attained age (age at death) on radiation carcinogenesis can now be examined.

As a reassessment of A-bomb dosimetry is currently under way, the shape of the dose response curve for gamma rays or the relative biological effectiveness (RBE) of neutrons based on the current A-bomb dosimetry system (tentative 1965 dose(T65D)) may change. Therefore, results of analyses of dose response and RBE based on the interim revised shielding dose estimates will also be introduced in this paper.

Study Sample

The LSS sample consists of persons who were living in either Hiroshima or Nagasaki at the time of the census of A-bomb survivors conducted by the Japanese government in 1950, five years after the bombing. As originally defined, the sample included 1) most persons who were within 2,500 m of ground zero in either city ATB, 2) a sample of persons who were between 2,500 and 10,000 m from ground zero, and 3) a sample of persons who were not in the city (NIC) or beyond 10,000 m ATB. The latter two samples were matched by city, sex, and age to a core group of survivors who were less than 2,000 m from ground zero ATB. The distribution of the total of 120,132 persons in the LSS sample by radiation dose and city is shown in Table I.

It has been observed that mortality in the NIC group is lower than that observed among survivors who were in the city ATB but received little or no radiation dose (the distally exposed group). It is generally believed that these differences in mortality are

TABLE I. Number of Subjects of the Extended LSS Sample

City	Total	Nonexposed	T65 dose in rad					
			0	1–9	10–99	100–199	200+	Unknown
Hiroshima	82,064	20,168	27,569	15,931	13,692	1,740	1,538	1,426
Nagasaki	38,068	6,349	15,397	7,137	5,470	1,388	1,369	958
Total	120,132	26,517	42,966	23,068	19,162	3,128	2,907	2,384

Source: Kato and Schull (*16*).

due to factors other than radiation exposure. For this reason the most recent analyses of LSS data have excluded the NIC group.

Ascertainment of Survival Status and Causes of Death

A family registration system (Koseki) was established in Japan about 100 years ago, under which all vital events which affect a family composition such as birth, death, and marriage are registered at the legal address (Honseki) of the family. Therefore, it is possible to ascertain easily and accurately the survival status of a study subject by checking the Koseki (Honseki) regardless of the actual residence of the person. Ascertainment of death is almost 100% complete in the LSS because the Koseki of the study subjects are checked periodically. Upon learning the fact of death and the address of the deceased as a result of the Koseki check, the cause of death is obtained from the vital statistics death schedule kept at the Health Center in which the address of the deceased is recorded. The vital statistics death schedules are prepared from death certificates, and thus the accuracy of the cause of death is a problem. In comparing the death certificate cause of death and that stated in the autopsy protocol, the latter diagnosis is treated as the true cause. Agreements or disagreements between the two sources of information can be examined in the following terms:

Principal autopsy diagnosis	Underlying cause of death		Total
	Disease X	Other than disease X	
Disease X	a Confirmed	b False negative	a+b
Other than disease X	c False positive	d Absence of disease	c+d
Total	a+c	b+d	a+b+c+d

Four possible outcomes are specified, two agreements (a and d) and two disagreements (b and c). The percentage of cases in which the underlying cause is confirmed by autopsy

TABLE II. Accuracy of Cause of Death for Malignant Neoplasms of Specific Sites, Autopsy Cases among the LSS Sample, 1961–75

Cause of death	Death certificate	Autopsy report	Agreement	Confirmation rate	Detection rate
Malignant neoplasms of:					
Buccal cavity and pharynx	19	17	13	68.4%	76.5%
Esophagus	50	53	36	72.0	67.9
Stomach	444	495	374	84.2	75.6
Large intestine	43	54	28	65.1	51.9
Rectum	45	46	32	71.1	69.6
Liver, gallbladder and bile duct	42	169	26	61.9	15.4
Pancreas	56	81	36	64.3	44.4
Trachea, bronchus, lung	192	172	117	60.9	68.0
Breast	40	49	38	95.0	77.6
Uterus	70	83	57	81.4	68.7
Prostate	13	24	5	38.5	20.8
Urinary organs	38	60	30	78.9	50.0
Malignant lymphoma	40	56	31	77.5	55.4
Leukemia	42	40	36	85.7	90.0

Source: Yamamoto *et al.* (*37*).

is called a confirmation rate, defined as 100a/(a+c). The complement of the confirmation rate, 100c/(a+c) is the false positive rate. Similarly, the rate of correspondence between the underlying cause of death and principal autopsy diagnosis is 100a/(a+b), termed the detection rate. Its complement, 100b/(a+b) is the false negative rate.

Table II shows the accuracy of the cause of death classification on death certificates as revealed by autopsy findings for those individuals who came to autopsy (*37*). Shown are the confirmation rate and detection rate by major cancer site. Confirmation and detection rates differ according to the cause of death: the rates are high for cancer such as leukemia, breast, and stomach, being over 70%, but the accuracy is poor for cancer such as the pancreas and liver where the confirmation rate is less than 50%. In studying cancer of sites having low accuracy, it is possible to restrict the study to only those that have been histologically confirmed either through autopsy or surgical pathology.

The underlying cause of death is classified according to the International Classification of Diseases (ICD). The cause of death has been coded by the 7th (1950–65), 8th (1968–78), and 9th (from 1979) revisions of the ICD.

Radiation Dose

The A-bombs dropped on Hiroshima (6 August 1945) and Nagasaki (9 August 1945) were of different design and content. A uranium bomb was used in Hiroshima and a plutonium bomb in Nagasaki. Whereas the radiation generated in Nagasaki consisted almost entirely of gamma rays, neutrons also contributed to the total dose received by survivors in Hiroshima; the amount, however, has recently become a matter of controversy and remains unresolved (*28*, *33*). The dose actually received by individuals differs according to their shielding; the shielding configuration and distance were established by interview for all members of the fixed samples. Their gamma ray and neutron kerma (tissue) doses, with consideration of the attenuation from shielding, were calculated in 1965; these dose estimates are referred to as T65D (*22*). The number of subjects in the sample by exposure dose is shown in Table I. Those exposed received a kerma dose of 27 rad on the average, but 6,000 individuals received a dose of 100 rad or more.

It must be borne in mind that uncertainty continues to surround both the quantity and quality of the radiation released by these two nuclear devices, particularly the Hiroshima bomb. Only one weapon of the Hiroshima type has ever been detonated and thus its yield has had to be reconstructed from tests and reactor experiments on other weapons. Different reconstructions have led to different estimates of the gamma ray and neutron exposure. A recent reassessment suggests that the gamma ray estimates used in the T65D calculations may be too low and the neutron estimates too high, and that the total kerma dose may have been greater than previously supposed (*21*), although another dosimetry review (*18*) differs in some of these particulars. This would have the effect of diminishing the slope of the dose-response curve based on total kerma and would make the results seen in the two cities more similar if these reassessments are correct. Given the uncertainties, attention here is restricted to exposure expressed as total kerma from the T65D estimates since this parameter changes least, relatively, for exposures of 10 rad or more when contrasted with the new dose assessments. Unfortunately, the new calculations are still too incomplete to form the basis of a meaningful dose-response analysis based upon individual exposure assessments. There are, for example, as yet no satisfactory estimates of building shielding factors or tissue attenuation of dose, although these estimates may be expected to change (*28*).

Statistical Methods

The statistical methods used here are described in detail elsewhere (*2*). Briefly, the exposed individuals in the sample (excluding the not-in-city and unknown dose groups) were divided into eight dose categories and a contingency table analysis was conducted adjusting for age ATB, sex, city, and period (year of death) using the Mantel-Haenszel method based on person-years at risk. In addition to the usual chi-square test, Cochran's linear trend chi-square test was calculated for the summary contingency table. Relative risks are defined as the ratios of two quotients, namely, the observed to expected deaths in the 100+ (or 200+) rad group and the observed to expected deaths in the 0 rad group where dose is the simple arithmetic sum of the estimated kerma from gamma rays and neutrons. The absolute risk was calculated from a linear regression of the excess deaths (observed / expected deaths) in each dose group in the summary contingency table using the mean for each dose group as the independent variable.

The cumulative death rates for specific cancer sites were calculated by the life table method considering the competing risk of death from other causes (*9*).

1. Cancer mortality by site

It is well known that the incidence rate of leukemia increased among A-bomb survivors. Mortality from malignant tumors other than leukemia also increased after a minimum incubation period of 10–15 years (*i.e.*, since 1955–60). However, this increase in cancer mortality was not observed for all cancer sites.

Mortality in the high dose group (200+ rad) for the period 1950–78 is presented in Fig. 1 by site as a relative risk based on mortality in the 0 rad group (*2*). A significantly elevated relative risk has been observed for leukemia and multiple myeloma, as well as for cancer of the esophagus, stomach, colon, lung, breast, and urinary tract. No elevation

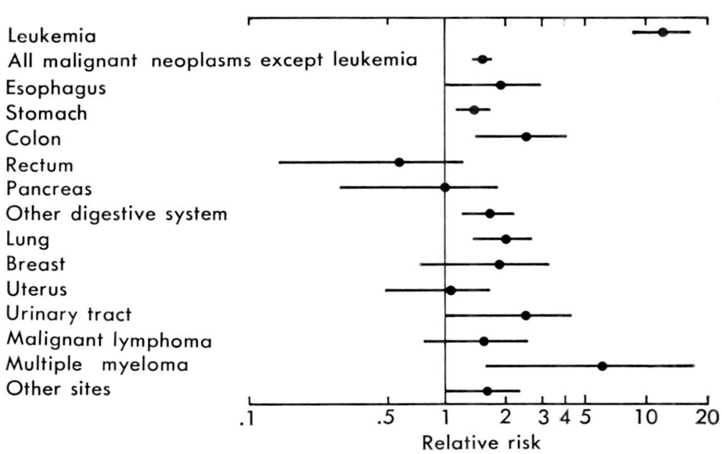

FIG. 1. Relative risk and 90% confidence intervals for specific cancer sites, 1950–78 (200+ rad *vs.* 0 rad).

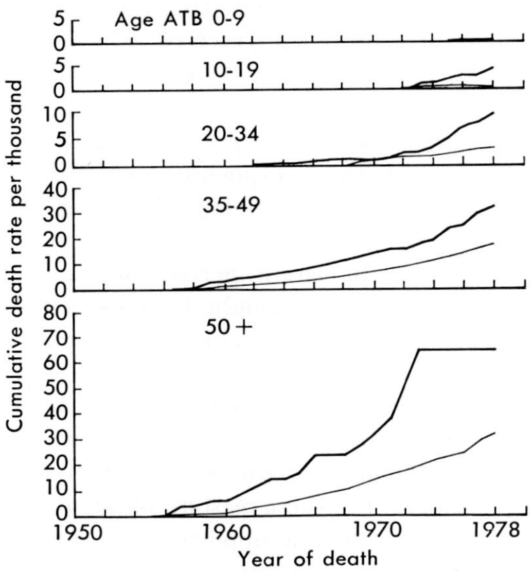

FIG. 3. Cumulative death rate per 1,000 (100+ rad (—) *vs*. 0–9 (—)) for lung cancer by age ATB, 1950–78.

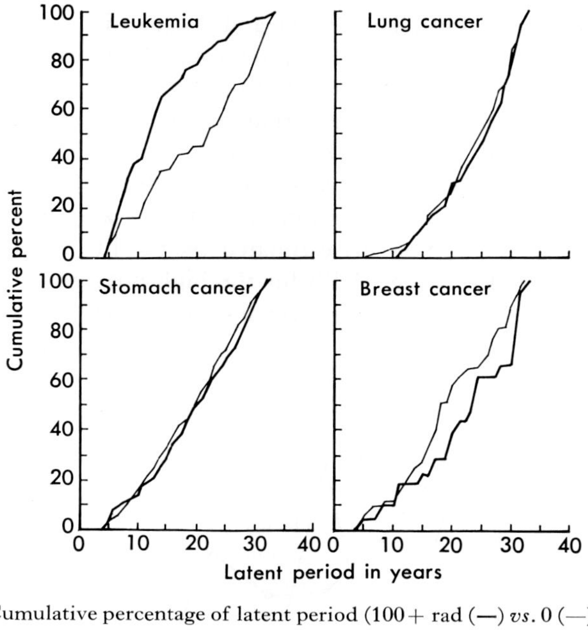

FIG. 4. Cumulative percentage of latent period (100+ rad (—) *vs*. 0 (—)) for specific cancer sites by radiation dose.

the high dose group according to age ATB: radiation-induced lung cancer develops only after the A-bomb survivors attain the age at which this cancer normally develops. This generally occurs at 40 or more years of age, and thus the period from A-bomb exposure to death (latent period) is longer the younger the age ATB. The same tendency is noted with breast and stomach cancer.

The distributions of the period until death for deaths due to leukemia and cancer of the stomach, lung, and breast are shown as cumulative percentages in Fig. 4 for the 100+ rad group and the 0 rad group (*16*). There is a dose dependent shortening of the latent period in leukemia (*20*) and, therefore, as the proportion of radiation-induced leukemia increased, the average period between exposure and death shortened, but this is not observed for stomach, breast, or lung cancer. Although not shown in Fig. 4, the latent period was not shortened for other solid tumors such as esophageal or colon cancer, collectively or by age ATB. The pattern of the latent period for malignant tumors induced by radiation differs for leukemia and malignant neoplasms other than leukemia. The reasons cannot be readily explained, but if an attempt is made to use the two-step mutational theory of carcinogenesis, or the theory that two factors, initiator and promoter, are generally necessary for the occurrence of cancer, it might be as follows:

For leukemia, the first and the second mutational steps necessary for radiation to cause transformation in cells may occur simultaneously or very nearly so, or in preconditioned individuals, (*i.e.*, those who have already undergone the first mutational step prior to exposure may be more numerous normally in human populations). Therefore, leukemia develops earlier the greater the exposure dose, irrespective of age ATB. For lung cancer, however, probably only the first mutational step is the result of exposure to radiation and the second and possibly other steps occur only when some other factor acts as a promoter. Cell transformation and proliferation then occur and the cancer develops. In this case, the time when the promoter acts to initiate the second step may be unrelated to the radiation dose, the initiator of the process. Hence, the latent period is unrelated to radiation dose and the cancer develops only when the age at which it is normally prone to develop is attained. Thus, the two different latency patterns can be explained by a two- (multi-) step mutational theory (*i.e.*, an initiator and a promoter are generally necessary in the induction of cancer) but with this alone the different latent patterns for chronic and acute leukemia cannot be explained (*20*). The changes in the immune response to irradiated cells have to be considered also, and in this sense the two-step hypothesis is open to the charge of overly simplifying the mechanism of radiation carcinogenesis, but it can be considered to be a reasonable working hypothesis to explain the differences in the patterns of latency.

Insofar as breast cancer is concerned, data other than those on A-bomb survivors have been reported recently from a study of this malignancy developing after X-ray therapy for postpartum mastitis (*29*) and from a study of the induction of breast cancer in tuberculosis patients following fluoroscopy of the chest (*5*). As with A-bomb survivors, no shortening of the latent period due to radiation dose was evident in either instance.

3. *Effects of age ATB and age at death*

As previously mentioned, radiation-induced solid cancers begin to appear after the age is attained at which the cancer is normally prone to develop, irrespective of age ATB. As shown in Fig. 5, there are two different models (relative risk and absolute risk models) that have been used to project a person's risk of death due to radiation induced cancer for their lifetime (*6*). The absolute risk model assumes that the excess deaths are constant by age at death throughout one's life, while the relative risk model assumes that excess deaths increase with age at death in proportion to age specific mortality rates of the control group; that is, the relative risks are constant by age at death throughout life.

As the estimated total number of excess deaths during a lifetime should be far

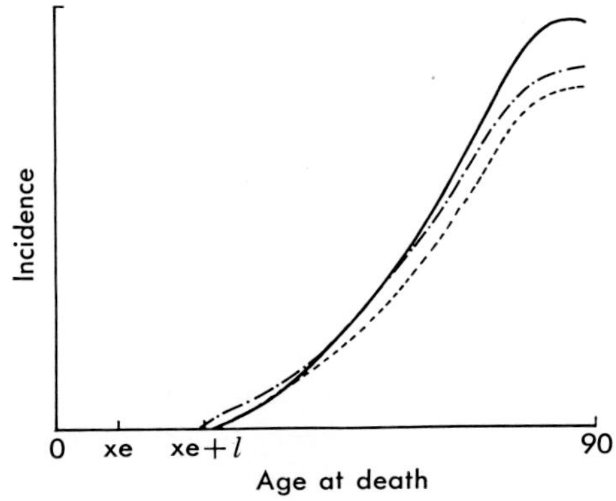

FIG. 5. Lifetime expression of radiation-induced cancer death rate: comparison of absolute (-•-) and relative (——) risk models. ----, spontaneous. Xe is age at exposure, l is the minimal latent period.

TABLE IV. Absolute Risk for All Cancer except Leukemia by Age ATB (Excess Deaths per 1,000,000 Person-year-rad (PYR)), 1950–78

Age ATB in years	Age at death in years					
	<30	30–39	40–49	50–59	60–69	70+
<10	1.22	4.35	13.41	—	—	—
10–19	0.03	1.72	4.62	20.69	—	—
20–34	—	1.35	1.01	7.97	10.25	—
35–49	—	—	0.26	−0.96	2.09	12.67
50+	—	—	—	17.39	0.53	18.31

Source: Kato and Schull (*16*).

larger under the assumptions of a relative risk model as compared with those of an absolute risk model, it is important to determine, if possible, which model fits best in a lifetime projection of the risk of radiation induced cancer.

The absolute risk (excess deaths per million person-year-rad (PYR)) of all cancer except leukemia (*16*) is shown in Table IV by six decades of age at death (<30, 30–, 40–, 50–, 60–, 70+) for specific age ATB groups (<10, 10–19, 20–34, 35–49, 50+). The excess deaths increase with age at death for the same age group in proportion to the age-specific death rate from cancer in the population of all Japan and do not show a constant excess value by age at death for the same age group. Thus the present data support the relative risk model projection more strongly.

Because radiation-induced cancer begins to appear after the age is attained at which the cancer is normally prone to develop, it is necessary to investigate the effect of age ATB on the estimation of the risk of radiation-induced cancer either adjusted or specific for age at death. The relative (200+ rad *vs.* 0 rad) and absolute risks of all cancer other than leukemia are shown by age ATB in Fig. 6, for the period 1950–78 (*16*). Age at death has not been considered. The relative risk is high in individuals of younger age ATB, although the absolute risk is higher with older ages ATB as would be expected. For age-at-death specific groups the relative risk for all cancer except leukemia (Table V) is higher the younger the age ATB. At the same age at death, the absolute risk is, like the relative risk, higher the younger the age ATB for all cancer other than leukemia

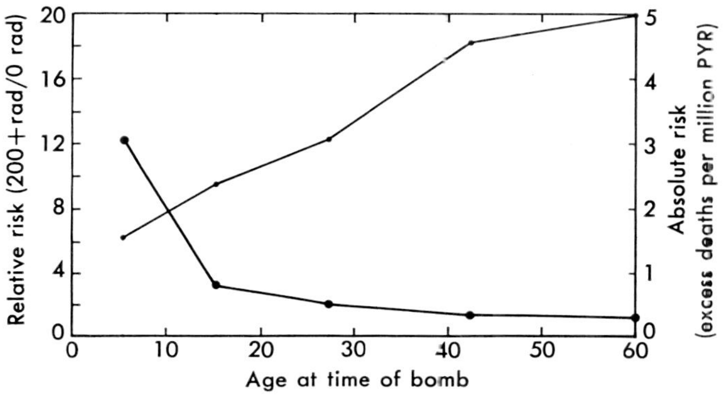

FIG. 6. Absolute risk (•) and relative risk (●) for all cancer except leukemia by age ATB.

TABLE V. Relative Risk for All Cancer except Leukemia by Age ATB, 100+ *vs.* 0 rad, 1950–78

Age ATB in years	Age at death in years					
	<30	30–39	40–49	50–59	60–69	70+
<10	15.1	5.0	6.8	—	—	—
10–19	1.0	2.5	2.4	8.2	—	—
20–34	—	1.8	1.9	2.0	1.6	—
35–59	—	—	1.2	1.1	1.3	1.4
50+	—	—	—	2.2	1.0	1.4

Source: Kato and Schull (*16*).

(Table IV). The tendency is similar or becomes much clearer if the value of the highest age ATB in each of the attained age classes (Table IV) is excluded (*i.e.*, assuming a minimum incubation period of 15 years). Thus, the higher absolute risk of radiation-induced cancer with advancing age ATB (Fig. 6) may be a deceptive phenomenon which has occurred because radiation-induced cancer has not increased appreciably in those who were young ATB and have not yet reached the ages at which the cancer develops.

The same tendency was also observed for other sites of solid tumors such as cancer of the lung, breast, and stomach. Thus, the effect of age ATB and the attained age has to be considered in estimating the risk of induction of cancer by radiation in man and it is difficult at present to estimate accurately the magnitude of the risk during a person's lifetime from the magnitude of the risk observed in A-bomb survivors. Survivors exposed at younger ages and their cancer experiences will have to be followed for some time.

Thus far, there are two exceptions to the general tendency described previously that the risk is higher in the younger age ATB group. One is that the incidence of cancer including leukemia during childhood did not increase among children exposed to A-bomb radiation while in utero (*13*). This finding does not support the results reported by Stewart and Kneale (*30*) that the incidence of childhood cancer increased among children whose mothers received diagnostic X-ray while pregnant. However, since the number of subjects in the RERF sample is small (only 2,600) follow-up of this sample is continuing. The results of follow-up until 1980 are shown in Table VI. The relative risk of cancer became high in the highest tissue dose (70+ rad) group, but an increasing

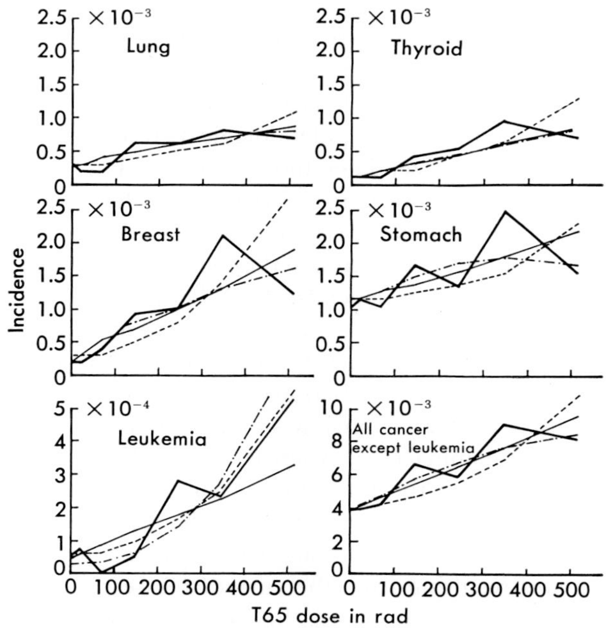

FIG. 7. Observed and expected average annual incidence of selected cancer sites, 1959–78. —, observed; ——, linear model; ----, quadratic; —•—, linear-quadratic.

The Q model fits better than the L or L-Q model for leukemia and the quadratic term of the L-Q model shows a positive value, though it is not statistically significant. On the contrary, the Q model does not fit and the L or L-Q model fit equally well for the incidence data of all cancer except leukemia. The linear term is significant in the L-Q model, whereas the quadratic term is not significant. Thus, this strongly suggests that the linear model fits best for all cancer except leukemia. A similar tendency was observed for specific cancer sites (lung, breast, thyroid, and stomach); the Q model either does not fit (for breast cancer) or fits more poorly than the L or L-Q model and the quadratic term in the L-Q model does not differ significantly from zero (the calculated value is negative).

Thus, it seems reasonable to use the linear model in risk estimation as has been done in the present analysis, though we cannot, statistically, distinguish one model from another among these three models except for cancer other than leukemia and breast cancer. In the dissenting section in the BEIR III report, Rossi (*27*) stated that the dose-response curve should be nonlinear and mortality from all cancer in Nagasaki for 1950–74 (*16*) fits a quadratic model best. The present analysis does not support this. Rather, the data suggest a linear model (see comments of Radford (*26*) in the same dissenting section) or at least a linear-quadratic model which the BEIR III committee used as the basis of risk estimation.

5. Estimation of the excess deaths from cancer among A-bomb survivors

It is important to place the risks cited in a larger public health perspective and to express the impact of radiation-related malignancies in relation to mortality in the general

TABLE IX. Estimated Number of Excess Cancer Deaths and Proportion to All Causes and Specific Cancer Site, 1950–78 (LSS Extended Sample, Exposed)

Cancer site	Excess deaths (90% confidence interval)			Upper: % to all causes Lower: % to specific causes			Death		
	Cities combined	Hiroshima (H)	Nagasaki (N)	H+N	H	N	H+N	H	N
Leukemia	90.6 (82.7–98.5)	66.36 (59.78–73.24)	27.31 (22.58–32.04)	0.39 50.3	0.36 47.1	0.54 70.0	180	141	39
All except leukemia	159.7 (120.7–198.7)	135.22 (102.66–167.77)	27.31 (4.09–50.74)	0.68 3.5	0.73 3.7	0.54 3.0	4,576	3,659	917
Esophagus	8.4 (1.1–15.8)	10.64 (4.38–16.90)	−2.15 (−6.45–2.15)	0.04 5.4	0.06 8.4	−0.04 −7.2	156	126	30
Stomach	41.6 (17.9–65.3)	31.61 (10.96–51.96)	10.32 (−3.23–24.08)	0.18 2.4	0.17 2.2	0.21 3.3	1,754	1,443	311
Colon	15.8 (8.4–22.7)	14.09 (8.14–20.35)	1.94 (−1.72–5.59)	0.07 10.1	0.08 10.6	0.04 8.1	157	133	24
Other digestive	24.2 (9.5–38.5)	20.03 (8.76–31.61)	4.52 (−5.16–13.98)	0.10 4.1	0.11 4.5	0.09 3.0	595	444	151
Lung	32.1 (19.5–45.3)	25.98 (15.65–36.31)	7.31 (−0.86–15.48)	0.14 7.0	0.14 7.4	0.15 6.9	459	353	106
Breast (Female)	15.4 (8.9–22.2)	12.88 (7.36–18.22)	2.83 (−1.23–7.01)	0.13 12.0	0.14 12.9	0.12 10.1	128	100	28
Urinary tract	7.9 (2.1–13.7)	4.70 (−0.31–9.70)	2.80 (−0.22–5.81)	0.03 7.6	0.03 5.2	0.06 20.0	104	90	14
Multiple myeloma	5.8 (2.6–8.4)	2.82 (1.25–4.70)	2.80 (0.65–4.95)	0.02 29.0	0.02 23.5	0.06 35.0	20	12	8

	Deaths from all causes	Mean dose	Average person-years	Subjects	Population at risk (10^6 PYR)
H+N	23,502 (11,740)[a]	27.2	24.27	79,856 (46,630)[a]	52.7×10^6 (30.8×10^6)[a]
H	18,471 (9,315)[a]	21.3	24.27	60,482 (35,607)[a]	31.3×10^6 (18.4×10^6)[a]
N	5,031 (2,425)[a]	45.8	24.27	19,374 (11,023)[a]	21.5×10^6 (12.3×10^6)[a]

[a] For female.

Source: Kato and Schull (*16*)

population. This assessment of excess deaths from cancer has been made, first, for the 79,856 A-bomb survivors who are the subjects of the analysis and, second, for all A-bomb survivors for the period 1950–78. Clearly, in both instances, the impact, at least in absolute terms, depends upon the population at risk, their exposure dose and years at risk, and the excess deaths per million PYR at risk. The average exposure dose among the subjects is 27.2 rad, and the average number of years at risk is 24.27. Thus, the population at risk is 52.7 million PYR ($79{,}856 \times 27.2 \times 24.27$). The excess deaths from cancer per million PYR are calculated for individual cancer sites assuming a simple linear dose-response relationship (*16*). The excess number of deaths from cancer is merely the population at risk multiplied by the excess deaths from cancer per million PYR; this excess for individual sites of cancer is shown in Table IX. The excess cancer deaths are also given in terms of their proportion of all causes of death and of deaths from individual cancer sites.

The 90.6 excess deaths from leukemia account for 50.6% of all leukemia deaths in this sample. For all cancer except leukemia, as a contrast, only 3.5% of the 4,575 such deaths in this sample are attributable to A-bomb radiation. This proportion, however, varies by site; from 29.0% for multiple myeloma to 2.4% for cancer of the stomach. In addition, 0.39% and 0.68% of the 23,499 deaths from all causes in this sample are attributable to A-bomb radiation for leukemia and all cancer except leukemia, respectively. These estimates are all based on the assumption of a linear increase with dose. The estimated number of excess deaths under the linear-quadratic model differ slightly; 62.2 and 208.5 for leukemia and cancer other than leukemia (corresponding to 34.7% and 4.6% deaths in the sample, respectively).

Among the 283,498 A-bomb survivors in all Japan enumerated at the time of the 1950 national census (mean exposure dose estimated to be 16.1 rad), it is estimated that 190.6 died of leukemia induced by A-bomb radiation and as many as 335.7 died of all cancer except leukemia. These estimates are for deaths occurring in the period 1950–78, and while hardly any increase can be expected for leukemia hereafter, deaths from cancer other than leukemia can be expected to increase in the future as the subjects attain the age at which such cancer is prone to develop. Therefore, at present it is difficult to estimate the number that would occur in the lifetime of the A-bomb survivors as a whole. From this point of view, these estimates do not go beyond merely providing a guide.

6. *Relationship between radiation and other carcinogenic factors*

A-bomb survivors have been exposed not only to radiation but also to other carcinogenic factors. It is essential, therefore, to ascertain whether the effect of radiation interacts with those of other carcinogenic factors, such as smoking. Such investigations may clarify the mechanism of radiation carcinogenesis. Data concerning factors other than radiation have been collected on this fixed population since 1960 through mail surveys, interview studies, and the national census. Several analyses have been conducted using these data. One example is the relationship between radiation exposure and principal occupation of the household head (a socioeconomic indicator) and breast cancer mortality. Shown in Fig. 8 is the mortality rate due to cancer of the breast for 1960–78 in the LSS sample (*16*) by radiation exposure and occupation. The age-adjusted breast cancer mortality rate is higher with higher socioeconomic status in both the 100+ rad group and the 0–9 rad group, and within each of the three socioeconomic classes, mortality in the 100+ rad group is increased about the same as in the 0–9 rad group. In other words,

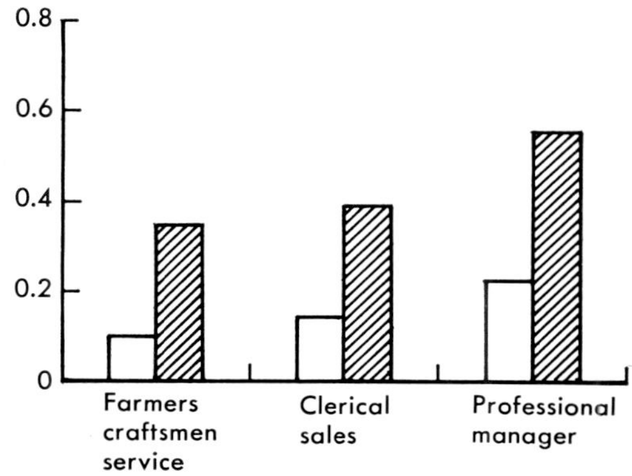

FIG. 8. Radiation and occupation, breast cancer, 1960–78. □, 0–9 rad; ▨, 100+ rad.

TABLE X. Number of Cases and Controls and Relative Risk for Lung Cancer according to Radiation Dose and Smoking Status

Sex	Smoker	Case/control	T65 dose in rad		
			0–9[a]	10–99	100+
Male	No[b]	Case	6 (1.0)[c]	3 (2.1)	4 (6.2)
		Control	74	21	9
	Yes	Case	130 (9.7)	38 (7.6)	26 (14.0)
		Control	240 (1.0)	100 (0.78)	34 (1.4)
Female	No	Case	62 (1.0)[c]	18 (0.7)	19 (5.3)
		Control	165	68	16
	Yes	Case	27 (2.0)	9 (2.1)	8 (4.5)
		Control	42 (1.0)	21 (1.1)	6 (2.3)

[a] Excludes persons not-in-city at the time of the bomb.
[b] These individuals were reported to have never smoked cigarettes.
[c] Reference category for relative risk is nonsmoking lightly exposed individuals. Relative risk given in parentheses is the odds ratio from logistic analysis for matched data run separately for males and females.
Source: Blot *et al.* (*4*).

there is no evidence of an interaction between radiation and household occupation (*i.e.*, they act additively).

Along the same line the Cox regression method, a multivariate statistical technique, was utilized to analyze cancer mortality in the LSS sample in relation to the joint effects of radiation dose and cigarette smoking habits as obtained by epidemiologic survey (*24*). Analyses were directed at all nonhematologic cancer and cancer of the lung, stomach, and other digestive organs. For all of these sites except lung, results support a submultiplicative relative risk model; that is, the relative risk for joint exposure to radiation and cigarette smoking is less than the product of the two individual relative risk estimates. This is particularly evident for those under 30 at the time of radiation exposure. In addition, there is suggestive evidence that the joint relative risk function for these sites may, indeed, be subadditive as well. The lung cancer relative risk function could not be distinguished from either a multiplicative or additive form, although there may be a slight preference for the additive model.

Similarly, a case control study of lung cancer has been conducted using 485 cases and 1,089 controls among LSS members during the period 1971–80. Results of preliminary analyses (*4*) suggest that A-bomb radiation and smoking combine in an additive manner to increase lung cancer risk as shown in Table X. This is in contrast to the multiplicative synergism between alpha radiation from radon and smoking reported among uranium miners (*36*).

7. Cancer mortality for early entrants

As described in detail elsewhere, numerous individuals included in the not-in-city group of the LSS sample entered Hiroshima or Nagasaki soon after the bomb for relief or other activities. If early entrants are defined as individuals who entered the city within one month after the bomb, 4,512 (3,698 in Hiroshima and 814 in Nagasaki) are included in the sample. These early entrants can be divided into three groups, a, b, and c, graded with respect to their estimated induced radiation dose, based on date and place of entry (Table XI). The cancer mortality of these groups during the period 1950–78 was compared with the not-in-city group other than early entrants (22,006 late entrants and the 31,581 subjects in the 0 rad group) (*16*).

Six deaths due to leukemia (4 in Hiroshima and 2 in Nagasaki) were recorded among early entrants during the entire survey period (Table XI). Leukemia mortality in this group, however, was lower than in the 0 rad group, but the difference is not statistically significant. Leukemia did not develop among the early entrants during the period 1950–58 when it was frequently occurring in the exposed groups, but developed later.

For all cancer except leukemia, mortality for the early entrants is lower than for the 0 rad group, and no significant difference is observed between early and late entrants although the latter are closer to the 0 rad group. Neither is there evident any difference in mortality between the three groups of early entrants (Table XI). By cancer site, mortality for early entrants for stomach, lung, and breast cancer is not significantly different from that for late entrants and the 0 rad group.

It is difficult to estimate precisely the dose of induced radiation received by early entrants. The mean cumulative dose from the bomb to infinite time is estimated to be no more than 2–3 rad in Hiroshima and considered to be less than 1 rad and negligible in Nagasaki (*10*). Thus, in view of the magnitude of the exposure dose and the fact that the irradiation of early entrants was chronic and not acute as in exposure to A-bomb

TABLE XI. Observed and Expected Deaths from Leukemia and All Cancer except Leukemia among Early Entrants, Late Entrants, and Exposed (0 rad)

Cancer site	Year	Statistic	Exposed (0 rad)	Early entrants	Late entrants	Test[a]	
						1	2
Leukemia	1950–78	0	40	6	11	*	*
		O/E	1.323	1.134	0.512		
All except leukemia	1950–78	0	1,654	276	1,041	*	NS
		O/E	1.025	0.900	0.992		

[a] Two tail test: 1, Exposed (0 rad) *vs.* total not-in-city (EE+LE); 2, Early entrants (EE) *vs.* late entrants (LE).

* Significant at 5% level.

NS, Not significant ($p>0.10$).

Source: Kato and Schull (*16*).

radiation, a remarkable increase in radiation-induced cancer seems highly unlikely as contrasted with directly exposed individuals.

There is one report which suggests an increase in the incidence of leukemia among early entrants (*11*, also published in Refs. *31*, *35*). However, there are some uncertainties: 1) the data are based on A-bomb handbook holders who are given free medical care and so will be biased towards inclusion of more leukemia cases; and 2) the population at risk was estimated based on three cross-sectional surveys conducted from 1950–74 and migration was not take into account.

It was recently reported that mortality from leukemia and other cancer increased among early entrants during 1968–72 based on an analysis of a sample of A-bomb handbook holders in Hiroshima prefecture (*19*). As this study is based on A-bomb handbook holders, it should also be affected by similar uncertainties due to the possible bias mentioned above. On the other hand, the RERF LSS data are based on a well-defined sample, but the number of early entrants in the sample was small. Further long-term follow-up is necessary.

8. An estimate of risk coefficient based on interim revised shielding dose estimates

As mentioned earlier, a reassessment of A-bomb radiation dosimetry is in progress by the committees appointed by the governments of Japan and the United States (*28*, *33*). However, because the revised dose system is not yet available, a tentative analysis (*7*) was conducted using interim shielding dose estimates as a trial.

Interim shielding dose estimates were tentatively calculated for 75,183 survivors belonging to the LSS, utilizing free-in-air dose curves by Pace and Scott of Oak Ridge National Laboratory (ORNL) and shielding factors developed by Marcum of R & D Associates (*18*). Deaths from leukemia and from all cancer sites except leukemia, chromosomal aberrations, and epilation were used as biological indices for assessing the effects of radiation as measured by these ORNL and T65D doses. Results thus obtained are as follows:

1. The Hiroshima and Nagasaki intercity differences in the dose-response are smaller for ORNL than that for T65D, but the risk is still higher for Hiroshima than for Nagasaki.

2. The estimated risk coefficients for gamma rays based on a linear model for both gamma rays and neutrons are larger for ORNL than for T65D for each effect, and the ratios of coefficients (ORNL *vs*. T65D) are in the range of 1.2 to 1.7.

3. As the ORNL neutron dose becomes very small even in Hiroshima, estimates of risk coefficients for ORNL neutrons may not be warranted. However, similar estimates as for gamma rays suggest that the risk coefficients are larger for ORNL than for T65D and ORNL/T65D ratios are in the range of 4–6. The estimated RBE for neutrons using ORNL dose and the linear model indicate that the RBE values for neutrons are larger for the ORNL dose than that for the T65D dose.

The results shown here are based on house-shielding dose tentatively estimated. Similar analysis based on organ dose tentatively estimated is under way. Final results of the effects of revising the A-bomb dosimetry must await the availability of the authorized A-bomb dosimetry system.

REFERENCES

1. Asano, M., Kato, H., Yoshimoto Y., Seyama, S., Itakura, H., Hamada, T., and Iijima, S. Primary liver carcinoma and liver cirrhosis in atomic bomb survivors, Hiroshima and Nagasaki, 1961–75, with special reference to hepatitis B surface antigen. *J. Natl. Cancer Inst.*, **69**, 1221–1227 (1982).
2. Beebe, G. W., Kato, H., and Land, C. E. Studies of the mortality of A-bomb survivors. 6. Mortality and radiation dose, 1950–74. *Radiat. Res.*, **75**, 138–201 (1978).
3. Beebe, G. W. and Usagawa, M. The Major ABCC Samples. ABCC Tech. Rep. 12-68 (1968).
4. Blot, W. J., Akiba, S., and Kato, H. Ionizing radiation and lung cancer; A review including preliminary results from a case-control study among A-bomb survivors. Proceedings of SIMS conference "Atomic bomb survivor data: utilization and analysis," Alta, Utah, September 12–16 (1983).
5. Boice, J. D., Jr. and Monson, R. R. Breast cancer in women after repeated fluoroscopic examinations of the chest. *J. Natl. Cancer Inst.*, **59**, 823–832 (1977).
6. Division of Medical Sciences, Assembly of Life Sciences, National Research Council, National Academy of Sciences. The effects on population of exposure to low levels of ionizing radiations 1979. Report of the Committee on Biological Effects of Ionizing Radiation (BEIR Report 3) (1980). NAS-NRC, Washington, D.C.
7. Fujita, S., Awa, A. A., Pierce, D. A., Kato, H., and Shimizu, Y. Re-evaluation of biological effects of atomic bomb radiation by changes of estimated dose. Proceedings of Symposium "Biological Effects of Low-level Radiation," Venice, 11–15 April, pp. 55–60 (1983). International Atomic Energy Agency, Vienna.
8. Fujita, S., Shimizu, Y., Masaki, K., Yoshimoto, Y., and Kato, H. RBE of neutrons in cancer mortality among atomic bomb survivors, Hiroshima and Nagasaki, 1950–78. RERF Tech. Rep. 9-80 (1980).
9. Gross, A. J. and Clark, V. A. "Survival Distributions: Reliability Applications in the Biomedical Science" (1975). Wiley, New York.
10. Hashizume. T., Maruyama, T., Kumamoto, Y., Kato, Y., and Kawamura, S. Estimation of gamma-ray dose from neutron induced radio-activity in Hiroshima and Nagasaki. *Health Phys.*, **17**, 761–771 (1969).
11. Hirose, F. Leukemia in atomic bomb survivors Hiroshima, 1946–1967. *Acta Haematol. Jpn.*, **31**, 765–771 (1968).
12. Ichimaru, M. and Ishimaru, T. Review of thirty years study of Hiroshima and Nagasaki atomic bomb survivors. II. Biological effects. D. Leukemia and related disorders. *J. Radiat. Res.* (Suppl.), **16**, 89–96 (1975).
13. Jablon, S. and Kato, H. Childhood cancer in relation to prenatal exposure to A-bomb radiation. *Lancet*, **2**, 1000–1003 (1970).
14. Kato, H. Host factor of cancer induction—with special reference to radiation carcinogenesis. *Byotai-Seiri*, **1**, 927–932 (1982) (in Japanese).
15. Kato, H., Brown, C. C., Hoel, D. G., and Schull, W. J. Studies of the mortality of A-bomb survivors, 7. Mortality, 1950–1978: Part II. Mortality from causes other than cancer and mortality in early entrants. *Radiat. Res.*, **91**, 243–264 (1982).
16. Kato, H. and Schull, W. J. Studies of the mortality of A-bomb survivors, 7. Mortality, 1950–1978: Part I. Cancer Mortality. *Radiat. Res.*, **90**, 395–432 (1982).
17. Kato, H. and Shigematsu, I. Late effects of A-bomb radiation, Hiroshima and Nagasaki. Effects of Nuclear War on Health and Health Services, pp. 117–138 (1984). World Health Organization, Geneva.
18. Kerr, G. D. (ed) Review of dosimetry for the atomic bomb survivor. The Fourth Sym-

posium on Neutron Dosimetry, Gesellschaft für Strahlen-und Umweltforschung, Munich-Neuherberg, June 1–5 (1981).

19. Kurihara, M., Munaka, M., Hayakawa, N., Yamamoto, H., Ueoka, H., and Ohtaki, M. Mortality statistics among atomic bomb survivors in Hiroshima Prefecture, 1968–1972. *J. Radiat. Res.*, **22**, 456–471 (1981).
20. Land, C. E. and Norman, J. E., Jr. Latent periods of radiogenic cancer occurring among Japanese A-bomb survivors. *In* "Late Biological Effects of Ionizing Radiation," Vol. 1, Proceedings of Symposium, Vienna, 13–17 March, IAEA-SM-224/602, pp. 29–47 (1978). International Atomic Energy Agency, Vienna.
21. Loewe, W. E. and Mendelsohn, E. Revised estimates of dose at Hiroshima and Nagasaki, and possible consequences for radiation-induced leukemia. (Preliminary) Report D 80–14 (1980). Lawrence Livermore National Laboratory, California, U.S.A.
22. Milton, R. C. and Shohoji, T. Tentative 1965 radiation dose estimation for atomic bomb survivors, Hiroshima and Nagasaki. ABCC Tech. Rep. 1-68 (1968).
23. Pinkston, J. A., Wakabayashi, T., Yamamoto, T., Asano, M., Harada, Y., Kumagami, H., and Takeuchi, M. Cancer of the head and neck in atomic bomb survivors, Hiroshima and Nagasaki, 1957–76. *Cancer*, **48**, 2172–2178 (1981).
24. Prentice, R. L., Yoshimoto, Y., and Mason, M. W. Relationship of cigarette smoking and radiation exposure to cancer mortality in Hiroshima and Nagasaki. *J. Natl. Cancer Inst.*, **70**, 611–622 (1983).
25. Preston, D. L., Kato, H., Kopecky, K. J., and Fujita, S. Life Span Study, Report 10. Part I. Cancer mortality among atomic bomb survivors, 1950–82. RERF Tech. Rep. 1-86 (1986).
26. Radford, E. P. Statement concerning the current version of cancer risk assessment in the Report of the Advisory Committee on the Biological Effects of Ionizing Radiation (BEIR III committee). BEIR III Report, pp. 287–314 (1980). National Academy Press, Washington, D.C.
27. Rossi, H. H. Separate Statement-Critique of BEIR III. *In* "The Effects on Populations of Exposure to Low Levels of Ionizing Radiation, 1980," pp. 254–260 (1980). National Academy Press, Washington, D.C.
28. Second US-Japan joint workshop for reassessment of atomic bomb radiation dosimetry in Hiroshima and Nagasaki. Proceeding of a workshop held at Hiroshima, 8–9 November 1983 (1983). RERF, Hiroshima.
29. Shore, R. E., Hempelmann, L. H., Kowaluk, E., Mansur, P. S., Pasternack, B. S., Albert, R. E., and Haughie, G. E. Breast neoplasm in women treated with X-ray for acute postpartum mastitis. *J. Natl. Cancer Inst.*, **59**, 813–822 (1977).
30. Stewart, A. and Kneale, G. W. Radiation dose effects in relation to obstetric X-ray and childhood cancers. *Lancet*, **1**, 1185–1188 (1970).
31. Sztanyik, L. B. Late biological effects of A-bombing in Japan. *In* "Late Biological Effects of Ionizing Radiation," Vol. 1, Proceedings of Symposium, Vienna 13–17 March, IAEA-SM-224/602, pp. 61–70 (1978). International Atomic Energy Agency, Vienna.
32. Tokunaga, M., Land, C. E., Yamamoto, T., Asano, M., Tokuoka, S., Ezaki, H., and Nishimori, I. Incidence of female breast cancer among A-bomb survivors, Hiroshima and Nagasaki, 1950–1980. RERF Tech. Rep. 15-84 (1984).
33. US-Japan joint workshop for reassessment of atomic bomb radiation dosimetry in Hiroshima and Nagasaki. Proceeding of a workshop held at Nagasaki, Japan, 16–17 February, ed. Thompson, D. J. (1983). RERF, Hiroshima.
34. Wakabayashi, T., Kato, H., Ikeda, T., and Schull, W. J. Studies of the mortality of A-bomb survivors, Report 7. Part III. Incidence of cancer in 1959–1978, based on the tumor registry, Nagasaki. *Radiat. Res.*, **93**, 112–146 (1983).
35. Watanabe, S. Cancer and leukemia developing among A-bomb survivors. *In* "Handbuch

der allgemeinen pathologie. Geschwülste. Tumors I. Morphologie, Epidemiologie, Immunologie," ed. Grundmann, E., p. 461 (1974). Springer-Verlag, Berlin.

36. Whittemore, A. S. and McMillan, A. Lung cancer mortality among US uranium miners: a reappraisal. *J. Natl. Cancer Inst.*, **71**, 489–499 (1983).

37. Yamamoto, T., Moriyama, I. M., Asano, M., and Guralnick, L. Radiation Effects Research Foundation Pathology Studies, Hiroshima and Nagasaki, Report 4. The Autopsy program and the Life Span Study, January 1961–December 1975. RERF Tech. Rep. 18-78 (1978).

METHODS FOR STUDY OF DELAYED HEALTH EFFECTS OF A-BOMB RADIATION

Edward P. RADFORD, Dale PRESTON, and Kenneth J. KOPECKY
*Department of Epidemiology and Statistics, Radiation Effects Research Foundation**

Methods for studying the delayed health effects of ionizing radiation among atomic bomb (A-bomb) survivors have been evolving in recent years. The chief delayed effects of interest are malignant and benign tumors in a defined sample of 93,614 survivors who were in Hiroshima and Nagasaki at the time of the bombing within 10,000 m from ground zero; nearly 65% of this group were in Hiroshima. In addition, a group of children irradiated in utero has been under study. Cancer cases are being identified from the tumor registries in both cities, as well as by death certificate searches; increasing emphasis is being placed on incident cases as well as certain benign tumors, which have been shown to be radiation-related. Previous methods of analysis have generally been by a contingency table technique, in order to compare cancer incidence and mortality rates, and to produce summary measures of risk or descriptions of radiation dose-response relationships. Application of new methods of analysis has been greatly aided by the availability of improved computer resources, as well as development of sophisticated statistical techniques. Examples are the use of hazard rate procedures, with relative and absolute risk models fitted to the data. Potential dose-effect modifiers that can readily be investigated include sex, age at exposure, time since exposure, attained age, and smoking, for example. In addition, a number of case-control studies have been carried out to investigate effects of factors potentially confounding A-bomb radiation effects. In particular, medical radiation exposures have been evaluated.

The follow-up studies of survivors of the atomic bombing in Hiroshima and Nagasaki have now extended for nearly 40 years, the largest prospective human epidemiologic study yet undertaken. In defining the effects of low doses of ionizing radiation, the A-bomb survivor study is especially important because it involves a group of people of all ages and both sexes who were in reasonable health prior to radiation exposure. Moreover, although many people who were near ground zero in both cities received radiation doses well over 100 rad, a high proportion of these did not survive long after the bombing, and therefore the majority of those in the study population of survivors identified in 1950 were exposed to much lower doses. For this reason the average tissue dose for those exposed to 1 rad or more is less than 20 rad, and thus many results are especially relevant to effects of low doses of radiation.

There has been much controversy about interpretation of data from each of the two cities. The two bombs differed in type of nuclear fuel, configuration of the contain-

* Hijiyama Park 5-2, Minami-ku, Hiroshima 732, Japan.

ment, and method of achieving a critical mass at the time of detonation. Until recently it was thought that the type of radiation exposure in the two cities differed significantly, in that the Hiroshima uranium-235 bomb was believed to have a much higher proportion of high energy neutron exposure at ground level than the Nagasaki plutonium-239 bomb. The most recent reassessment of dosimetry (*24, 44*), however, has indicated that the distribution of high energy neutrons by distance from ground zero was very nearly the same in both cities. Although the free-in-air gamma ray doses continue to be proportionately somewhat higher in Nagasaki compared to Hiroshima at equivalent distances, the neutron component in both cities is now too small to provide any conclusive basis for ascribing differences between results in each city to the quality of radiation exposure. If, as now appears to be the case, there are no significant differences in the radiation effects between the cities with the new doses, then the data for the two cities should be combined with suitable adjustment for differences between the city-specific spontaneous (0 dose) rates. This is advantageous because it increases the precision with which dose-response modification by other factors can be estimated.

This discussion will be restricted to methods appropriate for investigating cancer in the Japanese study populations. Radiation-induced cancer is the principal delayed health effect observed in groups irradiated at whole-body doses well below the acute lethal dose of about 400 rad, and it is also the main focus of this monograph. While the chief emphasis in the studies thus far has been on malignant neoplasms, there is evidence that the risk of certain benign or asymptomatic occult tumors may show an increase with increasing radiation exposure (*36*). Thus methods of ascertaining benign tumors are important in addition to detection of malignant cancer. Moreover, determination of radiation induction of benign and malignant tumors may throw additional light on the process of human carcinogenesis.

The study of delayed health effects of the bombings in 1945 was developed largely since 1950, and has continued to the present. This period of time has corresponded with a great development of epidemiologic and biostatistical methodology, as techniques of analysis originally developed to investigate epidemics of acute infectious diseases have been improved and extended in their application to chronic diseases such as cancer. Moreover, interest in noninfectious environmental causes of disease has greatly increased, and methods of detecting such environmental factors have become more sophisticated. This evolution of methodologic approaches to study of environmental factors in disease has made available many analytical techniques that were not considered at the time the A-bomb survivor studies were initiated.

Equally important has been the postwar development of extremely versatile and powerful computer technologies, which now permit use of analytical methods well beyond the capability of those available in 1950. The effect of these dramatic developments on the A-bomb studies is to emphasize the importance of reevaluating the analytical methods being applied to the results. Such reevaluation, coupled with the new assessment of radiation dosimetry from the two bombs, has led to important new developments in the study of cancer in the A-bomb survivors, and has altered some of the previously held perceptions concerning risks of radiation-induced cancer.

Study Populations

The primary resource available at Radiation Effects Research Foundation (RERF) for assessment of long-term effects of ionizing radiation is the Life Span Study (LSS) sample; follow-up of this sample began in October 1950. The LSS sample consists of persons who were living in either Hiroshima or Nagasaki at the time of the census of A-bomb survivors conducted by the Japanese government in 1950. As originally defined, the sample included 1) most persons alive at that time who were within 2,500 m from ground zero in either city at the time of the bomb (ATB), 2) a sample of persons who were between 2,500 and 10,000 m from ground zero ATB, and 3) a sample of persons who were not in city (NIC) or beyond 10,000 m. The latter two samples were obtained by matching by sex and age to a group of survivors who were less than 2,000 m from ground zero in each city. The original sample has been extended, most recently in 1982 by the addition of approximately 11,400 distally exposed (2,500–10,000 m) Nagasaki residents for whom complete follow-up data are available. As currently defined, the LSS population contains 120,132 subjects, of whom 38,890 were deceased by the end of 1982. A detailed description of the sample is presented in Beebe and Usagawa (*6*) and Kato and Schull (*23*).

An important methodological problem, typical of many epidemiologic studies, has been to define an appropriate control population, with which health effects in those persons exposed to radiation can be compared. In particular, cancer rates have been found in Japan, as elsewhere, to vary considerably by location (*15*). Thus analyses which compare rates among exposed survivors to national or prefectural cancer rates are of limited value and require careful attention to the possibility of bias. Moreover, it has been observed for many sites that mortality and incidence rates of cancer in the NIC group differ from those observed among survivors who were in the city ATB but received little or no radiation dose from the bombs. These differences in mortality and incidence are thought to arise from factors other than radiation exposure (*4*). For this reason most recent analyses of the LSS data have excluded the NIC group, and depended on those whose radiation exposure is estimated as zero (or less than 0.5 rad) as the control (non-exposed) population. With the NIC group eliminated, the total study population is presently 93,614 (61,911 in Hiroshima and 31,703 in Nagasaki).

In addition to the LSS population, other groups have been identified for follow-up study in the two cities. Only one of these, a group of 3,643 children who were in utero ATB, is currently considered relevant to the study of radiation-related cancer risks. But another group of potential interest for cancer evaluation is the 76,819 children of men and women who were A-bomb survivors; this group is primarily under study for genetic effects of radiation.

An important subset of the LSS is the Adult Health Study (AHS) population, which has had extensive and continuing clinical evaluations beginning in 1958. This group was selected to include a high proportion of individuals exposed to high doses, and a random sample of survivors with lower doses. In 1958 a total of 19,962 persons were selected from the entire LSS population, as it was then defined. Of these, 16,738 had been examined at least once by the end of 1978 (*25*). In 1977, another 2,436 persons were added to the AHS population, and over 60% of these were examined at least once within four years (*36*). All AHS subjects living in or near either city are encouraged to return every two years for detailed evaluation of their health status, including medical history, physical examination, laboratory evaluations, and special clinical studies as needed. The participation rate has declined with successive examination cycles. By the 11th two-year cycle of examinations (July 1978–June 1980) over 30% of the original AHS sample had been lost due to death or migration out of the Hiroshima and Nagasaki contacting areas. However, among the remaining persons, and excluding the NIC group, the participation rate was rather high: the proportion of contactable persons actually examined was 70% in Hiroshima and 85% in Nagasaki (*36*). For members of the NIC group, who since 1975 have been contacted only by mail, the participation rate had fallen to only 41% in each city by the 11th cycle (*36*). Altogether 9,387 subjects (7,929 exposed and 1,458 NIC) were examined in that cycle.

Source of Data

The basic data available for each member of the LSS sample are city of residence, sex, and date of birth. For most exposed survivors there are also estimates of the gamma ray and neutron dose received. Those survivors with dose data unassigned numbered 2,386 in 1980, but this number is expected to increase with the adoption of a new dosimetry system. As of this writing the results of radiation dose reevaluations, for which there is fair agreement, indicate the following: 1) As mentioned above, neutron components of the total doses in both cities are so small and so similar that accurate estimation of a differential health effect of gamma rays and neutrons based on intercity comparisons is not feasible. 2) Gamma ray free-in-air doses in Hiroshima are higher by a factor of about 2 to 3 than the old tentative 1965 (T65) doses, while in Nagasaki the free-in-air gamma ray doses are now slightly lower than previously. 3) Shielding by buildings or terrain was much more effective in reducing gamma ray exposure than was thought previously, but shielding by body tissue was somewhat less effective. The net effect is that transmission factors, which are applied to free-in-air gamma ray dose to give tissue dose, are substantially reduced, especially in Nagasaki, where a relatively high percentage of survivors from whom shielding histories were obtained were in factories or shielded by terrain. 4) In comparison with the 1965 dosimetric evaluation (*30*), the new dosimetry indicates that total radiation doses will be reduced more in Nagasaki than in Hiroshima.

Data on mortality within the LSS sample is obtained by periodic checks of the Japanese system of local family registration offices (Honseki). These offices maintain records of family vital events, births, marriages, deaths, *etc.*, and each living sample member's record (Koseki) is periodically reviewed to determine vital status. Whenever a record of a person's death is found, the date and cause of death are obtained from the vital statistics death schedule at the Health Center for the place of death; the cause of death reported by these centers is obtained from death certificates. Because of the comprehensive nature of the Koseki system, ascertainment of death is believed to be virtually complete for subjects resident in Japan. The hazards of relying on death certificates to establish the primary cause of death are well known. A comparison of certified cause of death and autopsy diagnoses (*38*, *46*) revealed that cancer confirmation and detection rates vary widely according to the type of cancer. The accuracy of death certificates in the LSS population was found to be high for malignant neoplasms of some organs such as breast and stomach, and for leukemia. But for others, such as lung, urinary tract, liver and biliary system, pancreas, and prostate, death certificate data were found to underestimate the presence of cancer considerably (*35*). This underestimation will produce an equivalent underestimation of the absolute excess risks associated with exposure to radiation. In the AHS sample, ascertainment of cases includes a wide range of disease conditions studied in relation to radiation effects, but in this report we are concerned mainly with benign or malignant tumors.

Data on cancer incidence are also obtained through the tumor registries established in both cities by the local medical societies in the late 1950s, tissue registries in each city, and supplementary case finding efforts conducted for particular studies. At this time reporting of cases by the tumor registries is considered to be good for the two cities. The registries incorporate cases only for those resident in each city at the time of the diagnosis, thus there is underascertainment of cases in the LSS population because of migration out of the cities, a particular problem for those who were young ATB. Data from the AHS population indicate that since 1958 out-migration has been slight (only a few percent). However, prior to that time about 10% of all those living had left. As many as 20% of the members of the youngest age ATB groups may have left the cities prior to 1958. Tokunaga *et al.* (*42*) cited evidence that among AHS females the migration rate was unrelated to radiation dose. Because most of those leaving have settled in the large cities of Honshu and Kyushu, it is possible that they could be traced to tumor registries there, in order to bring the ascertainment of incident cancer closer to 100%.

The cancer incidence data have the advantage that cases are included in the study at the time of diagnosis, often years before fatal cancer would be found from death certificate records. Not only may there be a substantial lag between diagnosis and death, but sometimes as much as two years may elapse before the death certificate data are recorded and detected from the Koseki. The delay in ascertainment from death records is especially important because cancer cases in the LSS are rapidly accumulating, and the evidence of radiation dose-related effects is increasing.

Another important factor in use of tumor registry data is the fact that cases are recorded regardless of outcome. Thus information on nonfatal malignancies and some types of benign tumors can be obtained from the registries. This issue is especially significant for cancer of the thyroid and female breast, which are radiosensitive but not highly fatal. The radiosensitivity of cancer of the prostate is uncertain, in part because ascertainment of cases of cancer of the prostate from death certificates is poor in Japan. Data from the tumor registries, for which ascertainment is somewhat better, indicate a radiation dose-related effect (*43*). Finally, it should be emphasized that use of incident cancer as a basis of defining cancer risks gives an indication of radiation effects that is generally more meaningful in terms of total social cost than simply cancer deaths alone.

Ascertainment of benign tumors from the tumor registries evidently is somewhat incomplete, as judged by comparison with results obtained from the AHS examinations. Thus it may be that the latter group will yield the most definitive information on benign tumors. It is worth noting that in the AHS, radiation dose-related effects have been observed for nonmalignant thyroid disease, gastric polyps, and uterine fibromas, and in an autopsy study, precancerous breast lesions were also found to be radiation-related.

Confounding Factors

Data concerning host and environmental characteristics such as smoking habits, diet, socioeconomic status, childbearing history, occupation, and many other details have been collected in a series of interview and mail surveys of large subsets of the LSS sample conducted at various times between 1963 and 1981. These data have been useful in efforts to deal with factors other than A-bomb radiation exposure which might affect cancer risks. For example, smoking experience is important to take into account in lung cancer studies, as well as potentially for other smoking-related cancer. Smoking information is available from several of the surveys of the LSS population.

Another important potential confounding factor is exposure of the study population to medical X-rays. Evaluation of this source of additional radiation exposure could be important in future analyses of LSS data, particularly for those subjects given X-ray therapy for benign conditions. A survey of hospitals in the Hiroshima area, as well as among the AHS population, indicates that average cumulative radiation exposure to the bone marrow or gonads since 1945 has been less than 2 rad from diagnostic X-ray, although a few persons in the LSS population have accumulated doses over 20 rad (*37*). With regard to therapeutic radiation, local doses in excess of 1,000 rad have been received by approximately 2,000 persons in the LSS (*33*). About 65% of this therapy has been for cancer, therefore among this group the primary interest is in the possibility of second primary malignancies.

Previous Methods of Analysis of LSS Data

Studies of the effects of radiation exposure on mortality and disease incidence in the LSS involve the estimation and comparison of rates, to produce summary measures of risk or to provide detailed descriptions of radiation dose-response. The summary measures reported in most analyses of the LSS data are estimates of absolute excess risk or of relative risk. The absolute risk is the number of excess cases per person year (PY) per rad while the relative risk is the proportional increase in risk per rad. The results in the two cities are age-adjusted to the combined population. Most published analyses of morbidity in the sample have made use of the so-called contingency table method, which was originally developed by Land for a survey of mortality through 1966 (*4*), and has been used in a slightly modified form in the two recent surveys of mortality in the LSS (*5*, *23*), as well as in special studies of specific diseases, such as Ichimaru *et al.* (*20*) and Tokunaga *et al.* (*42*). This method has been described in detail by Preston (*34*). Briefly, statistics for heterogeneity of risk among dose categories are partitioned into sums of squares of asymptotically normal statistics. The latter statistics are simply regression coefficients obtained by the use of orthogonal contrasts designed to test particular alternative hypotheses of interest, an approach derived from Cochran (*11*). The alternative hypothesis of primary interest has usually been that the radiation-induced absolute excess risk, averaged over some follow-up period of interest, increased as a linear function of radiation exposure dose. The Mantel-Haenszel procedure (*28*, *29*) was employed to calculate expected number of deaths and covariance matrices, adjusting for differences between strata defined by city, sex, and age ATB. The contingency table method, as it has usually been applied in studies at RERF, is based on internal comparisons of mortality rates among exposed survivors. However, some reports (*21*, *31*) have made use of Japanese national death rates for the calculation of expected number of deaths.

The analyses in the various reports cited above were similar in several key respects: 1) In none of the reports were the analyses of trends in dose adjusted for temporal variation of background mortality rates during the period of follow-up. However, recent computations have shown that this adjustment leads to only minor changes in results of analyses of the LSS data. 2) As applied, the contingency table method provided only estimates and test statistics for the radiation dose-response parameter, but did not provide information for formally estimating the magnitude or testing the significance of dose effect modification by other factors. Therefore the comparison of the radiation dose-responses by city, sex, age ATB, or subinterval of follow-up had to be based on informal interpretations of the results of separate analyses for various subsets of the data. An untoward result of this was the necessity for an extremely large number of separate, but frequently correlated significance tests. 3) The observed levels of significance (p values) for the various statistical tests were all based on asymptotic chi-square and normal distributions. For many causes of death, the highly skewed distribution of the LSS sample with respect to radiation dose leads to quite small expected number of deaths in the high dose categories. It has been recognized that in this situation the normal-theory p values underestimate the true significance levels (*19*). Some reports have attempted to deal with this problem by employing fourth-order Edgeworth approximations of the trend statistic's sampling distributions (*5*, *42*).

Historically, retrospective studies have played a less important role than cohort studies for investigations of cancer among A-bomb survivors, although in recent years a number of case-control studies have been undertaken. These have included studies of cancer of the female breast (*45*), the lung (*7*), and colon and rectum (*1*). The procedures and statistical analyses which have been conducted or planned for these case-control studies are based on standard techniques (*9*) and will not be discussed in this paper.

Hazard Rate Models for the LSS Data

Recent advances in statistical and computational methodology have made it possible to introduce sophisticated and powerful new techniques for the analysis of large sets of survival data. These methods have been described by Cox (*13*), Kalbfleisch and Prentice (*22*), Lawless (*27*), and others. These new techniques, which make use of explicit models for the underlying hazard (instantaneous rate) function make it possible to study the temporal variation in the background and radiogenic components of the observed rates and to formulate and test specific hypotheses about modification of the dose-response by factors such as age ATB and sex. In this section several classes of hazard function models are discussed and some specific models which have proven useful in analyses of the LSS cancer data are described. Computational methods and software for parameter estimation, hypothesis testing, and the assessment of goodness-of-fit based on these models are also discussed briefly. The emphasis here is placed on the case in which there is a single, instantaneous exposure to the factor of primary interest. Thomas (*40*) and Gilbert (*18*) consider the use of hazard rate modeling methods in cases of prolonged exposure.

Let $\mu(t;\, \boldsymbol{z},\, d)$ denote the hazard function at time t for a person who received dose d; the vector $\boldsymbol{z}$ contains information about covariates other than radiation dose, such as city, sex, age ATB, smoking, *etc.* The hazard function corresponds to the incidence or mortality rate as a continuous function of time. Two simple models for the hazard function might be considered. In the first, a pure relative risk model, the relative risk is a function of dose only. Such a model can be written as

$$\mu(t;\, \boldsymbol{z},\, d) = \lambda(t;\, \boldsymbol{z})\rho(d)\,, \tag{1}$$

where $\lambda(t;\, \boldsymbol{z})$ denotes the natural or background rate of morbidity in the absence of radiation exposure, and $\rho(d)$ is the relative risk function. Similarly, one can define a purely additive excess risk model in which the excess risk for dose d does not depend on time or the other covariates:

$$\mu(t;\, \boldsymbol{z},\, d) = \lambda(t;\, \boldsymbol{z}) + \varepsilon(d)\,, \tag{2}$$

where $\varepsilon(d)$ is the additive excess risk function. Potentially more realistic models are obtained if we allow for dose-effect modification by the other factors. It is also important to consider more general hazard functions in which the relative and excess risk functions are allowed to vary with time. In their most general form these models can be written as

$$\mu(t;\, \boldsymbol{z},\, d) = \lambda(t;\, \boldsymbol{z})\rho(d;\, t,\, \boldsymbol{z}) \tag{3}$$

and

$$\mu(t;\, \boldsymbol{z},\, d) = \lambda(t;\, \boldsymbol{z}) + \varepsilon(d;\, t,\, \boldsymbol{z})\,, \tag{4}$$

in which case the distinction between relative and absolute risk models disappears. Useful models for the study of radiation effects lie somewhere between the extremes of the too-simple models (1) and (2) and the too-rich models (3) and (4). In analyses of RERF data based on hazard rate models, excess risks have generally proven to be time dependent. Absolute excess risk models which include such time dependence are generalizations of the standard absolute risk models which are discussed in the literature on radiation effects and which do not allow the excess risk to change in time after an initial latent period; see for example the 1980 BEIR Report (*12*), 169–172.

In studies at RERF, interest is centered on the dose-related relative or excess risk functions. Partial likelihood methods for relative risk models, as originally proposed by Cox (*13*) and discussed at length by Kalbfleisch and Prentice (*22*), allow one to focus on the estimation of the relative risk without the explicit estimation of the background hazard function $\lambda(t;\, \boldsymbol{z})$. It is sometimes of interest in relative risk models, and it is necessary for estimation in absolute excess risk models, to consider fully specified parametric models for the background rates (*i.e.*, the natural rates of mortality or disease incidence in the absence of exposure to radiation). The models used for background rates in current studies at RERF are generally log-linear models of the form exp $(\beta^* \boldsymbol{z}^*)$ where $\boldsymbol{z}^*$ includes not only variables related to city, sex, smoking, *etc.*, but also functions of attained age which replace the time-since-exposure variable t. Continuous or indicator functions of age ATB can be included to allow for secular trends in the rates.

Discussions of relative risk functions are often based on log-linear $(e\beta \boldsymbol{x})$ or additive $(1+\beta \boldsymbol{x})$ forms for the relative risk, where the vector $\boldsymbol{x}=x(d,\, \boldsymbol{z})$ can include both dose- and covariate-related components. A simple example of the former is β, while an example of the latter is given by $(1+\beta,\, \beta+\boldsymbol{z})$ where $\boldsymbol{z}$ is a potential dose effect modifier such as a function of age ATB.

Recently there has been interest in general relative risk models which can be used to discriminate between multiplicative and additive relative risks. Aranda-Ordaz (*2*) and Breslow (*8*) have suggested the use of relative risk functions of the form

$$l(\rho(\boldsymbol{x})) = [(1+\beta \boldsymbol{x})^{\delta} - 1]/\delta \tag{5}$$

This class of relative risk models includes both the multiplicative and additive models as special cases; $\delta=1$ for the multiplicative and the limit as δ goes to 0 for the additive model. Thomas (*41*) has suggested an alternative approach to this problem.

The excess risk models used thus far in analyses of the A-bomb survivor data have the form

$$\varepsilon(d, \boldsymbol{z}) = \phi(d)\omega(\boldsymbol{z}, t)$$

where the $\phi(d)$ is typically linear in dose and $\omega(t, \boldsymbol{z})$ is log-linear in various functions of the covariates and time. The function $\phi(d)$ can be thought of as a baseline dose-response while the function $\omega(t, \boldsymbol{z})$ allows for deviations from this baseline dose-response due to characteristics of the individuals or the passage of time. While the baseline dose-response can be linear, one could easily consider nonlinear functions of total dose.

Methods of Estimation for Hazard Rate Models

Likelihood methods are used for parameter estimation and hypothesis testing with hazard rate models. A few analyses have been carried out using the full likelihood for the ungrouped data. Such analyses have been done primarily to compare the resulting parameter estimates and their standard errors with those obtained when functionally identical models were fit to grouped data using the methods outlined below. Full likelihood methods are not practical for use with general, time-dependent hazard rate models such as those described above.

Partial likelihood methods for relative risk models have proven useful in the analysis of the RERF data. As noted above, this approach is appealing because it eliminates the need to model the background rates explicitly. Although partial likelihood methods cannot be used for absolute risk models, the inclusion of time-dependent covariates makes it possible to consider relative risks which are not constant in time. The major limitation of this approach is that it is computationally intensive. On a medium-sized mainframe computer (*e.g.*, NEC ACOS-450) over one hour of computer time is required to fit a relative risk model with time-dependent covariates to the LSS data.

Another approach to the analysis of large sets of survival data which overcomes the limitations of the methods discussed above makes use of grouped data. The ideas underlying the use of grouped data in the analysis of cohort studies have been described in several recent papers (*8*, *10*, *17*, *32*). As in the contingency table analysis described above, the basic data are the number of cases or deaths, Y_{ijk}, and PY or number of persons at risk, P_{ijk}, together with a dose, d_{ij}, and vector of covariates, $\boldsymbol{z}_{ijk}$, associated with each cell in a cross-classification over city, sex, age ATB, and, perhaps, other factors (i), dose groups (j), and subintervals of follow-up (k). The components of $\boldsymbol{z}_{ijk}$ may be indicator variables or, for quantitative factors such as age, time, cigarette consumption, *etc.*, classmark values such as category-specific means or midpoints; the components of $\boldsymbol{z}_{ijk}$ may also include cross-products involving dose. If the P_{ijk} are regarded as fixed and the risk per unit time is considered to be a constant, μ_{ijk}, within each cell of the cross-classification, then the kernel of the likelihood function is identical to that which would arise if the Y_{ijk} are treated as independent Poisson random variables with mean $P_{ijk}\mu_{ijk}$. The parameters μ_{ijk} correspond to specific rates of incidence or mortality. For the purpose of modelling these rates, parametric or semiparametric models for the underlying hazard function can be considered. Maximum likelihood estimation and likelihood-based hypothesis tests are derived from the Poisson likelihood.

This approach has many advantages. First, it can be used to fit either relative risk or absolute excess risk models. The theory of likelihood-based inference provides a preliminary results from a case-control study among A-bomb survivors. *In* "Atomic Bomb Survivor Data: Utilization and Analysis," ed. R. L. Prentice and D. J. Thompson, pp. 235–248 (1984). SIAM, Philadelphia.

8. Breslow, N. E. Cohort analysis in epidemiology. University of Washington, Dept. of Biostatistics. Technical Report No. 65 (1984).
9. Breslow, N. E. and Day, N. E. "Statistical Methods in Cancer Research Volume 1—The Analysis of Case-control Studies (1980). IARC, Lyon.
10. Breslow, N. E., Lubin, J. H., Marek, P., and Langholz, B. Multiplicative models and cohort analysis. *J. Am. Stat. Assoc.*, **78**, 1–12 (1983).
11. Cochran, W. G. Some methods for strengthening the common x2 tests. *Biometrics*, **10**, 417–451 (1954).
12. Committee on the Biological Effects of Ionizing Radiation. The Effects on Populations of Exposure to Low Levels of Ionizing Radiation: 1980 (1980) National Academy Press, Washington, D.C.
13. Cox, D. R. Regression models and life tables (with discussion). *J. R. Stat. Soc. Ser. B*, **34**, 187–220 (1972).
14. Cox, D. R. and Hinkley, D. V. "Theoretical Statistics" (1974). Methuen, New York.
15. Daiwa Health Foundation. Atlas of cancer mortality for Japan by cities and counties, 1969–71, Tokyo, 1977.
16. Dempster, A. P., Laird, N. M., and Rubin, D. B. Maximum likelihood from incomplete data *via* the Em algorithm. *J. R. Stat. Soc. Ser. B.*, **39**, 1–38 (1977).
17. Frome, E. L. The analysis of rates using Poisson regression models. *Biometrics*, **39**, 665–674 (1983).
18. Gilbert, E. S. An evaluation of several methods for assessing the effects of occupational exposure to radiation. *Biometrics*, **39**, 161–171 (1983).
19. Hoel, D. G. and Jennrich, R. I. Life table analysis with small numbers of cases, an example multiple myeloma in Hiroshima and Nagasaki. RERF Tech. Rep. 9–84 (1984).
20. Ichimaru, M., Ishimaru, T., Mikami, M., Yamada, Y., and Ohkita, T. Incidence of leukemia in a fixed cohort of atomic bomb survivors and controls, Hiroshima and Nagasaki: October 1950—December 1978. RERF Tech. Rep. 13-81 (1981).
21. Jablon, S. and Kato, H. Studies of the mortality of A-bomb survivors. 5. Radiation dose and mortality, 1950–1970. *Radiat. Res.* **50**, 649–698 (1972).
22. Kalbfleisch, J. D. and Prentice, R. L. "The Statistical Analysis of Failure Time Data" (1980). Wiley, New York.
23. Kato, H. and Schull, W. J. Studies of the mortality of the A-bomb survivors. 7. Mortality 1950–1978, Part I. Cancer Mortality. *Radiat. Res.*, **90**, 395–432 (1982).
24. Kerr, G. D., Pace, J. V., III, and Scott, W. H., Jr. Tissue kerma *vs.* distance relationships for initial nuclear radiation from the atomic bombs, Hiroshima and Nagasaki (1983). *In* "Reassessment of Atomic Bomb Dosimetry," pp. 57–103. (1983) RERF, Hiroshima.
25. Kodama, K., Shimizu, Y., Sawada, H., and Kato, H. Incidence of stroke and coronary heart disease in the Adult Health Study sample, 1958–78. RERF Tech. Rep. 22-84 (1984).
26. Kopecky, K. J., Yamamoto, T., Fujikura, T., Tokuoka, S., Monzen, T., Nishimori, I., Nakashima, E., and Kato, H. Lung cancer, radiation exposure and smoking among atomic bomb survivors, Hiroshima and Nagasaki, 1950–1980. RERF Tech. Rep. in preparation.
27. Lawless, J. F. "Statistical Models and Methods for Lifetime Data" (1982). Wiley, New York.
28. Mantel, N. and Haenszel, W. Statistical aspects of the analysis of data from retrospective studies of disease. *J. Natl. Cancer Inst.*, **22**, 719–748 (1959).
29. Mantel, N. Chi-square tests with one degree of freedom: extensions of the Mantel-Haenszel procedure. *J. Am. Stat. Assoc.*, **58**, 690–700 (1963).

30. Milton, R. C. and Shohoji, T. Tentative 1965 radiation dose estimation for A-bomb survivors, Hiroshima and Nagasaki, ABCC Tech. Rep. 1-68 (1968).
31. Moriyama, I. M. and Kato, H. JNIH-ABCC Life Span Study, Report 7. Mortality experience of A-bomb survivors, 1950–72. ABCC Tech. Rep. 15-73 (1973).
32. Pierce, D. A., Preston, D. L., and Ishimaru, T. A method of analysis of cancer incidence in Japanese atomic bomb survivors with application to acute leukemia, RERF Tech. Rep. 15-83 (1983).
33. Pinkston, J. A., Antoku, S., and Russell, W. J. Malignant neoplasms among atomic bomb survivors following radiation therapy. *Acta Radiol. Oncol.*, **20**, 267–271 (1981). (Also personal communication, W. J. Russell, 1984).
34. Preston, D. L. Cancer mortality and incidence in the Life Span Study: statistical methods used in Reports Five through Ten. *In* "Atomic Bomb Survivor Data: Utilization and Analysis," ed. R. L. Prentice and D. J. Thompson, pp. 35–50 (1984). SIAM, Philadelphia.
35. Radford, E. P. A comparison of incidence and mortality as a basis for determining risks from environmental agents. *In* "Proc. of the 20th Annual Meeting of the National Council on Radiation Protection and Measurements," pp. 75–88 (1985). NCRP, Bethesda, Md.
36. Sawada, H., Kodama, K., Shimizu, Y., and Kato, H. RERF Adult Health Study Report 6: Results of six examination cycles, 1968–1980. Hiroshima and Nagasaki. RERF Tech. Rep., in preparation.
37. Sawada, W., Land, C. E., Otake, M., Russell, W. J., Takeshita, K., Yoshinaga, H., and Hombo, Z. Hospital and clinic survey estimates of medical x-ray exposures in Hiroshima and Nagasaki. Part I, RERF population and the general population. RERF Tech. Rep. 16-79 (1979).
38. Steer, A., Moriyama, I. M., and Shimizu, K. The autopsy program and the life span study, January 1951–December, 1970. ABCC Tech. Rep. 16-73 (1973).
39. Storer, B. E., Wacholder, S., and Breslow, N. E. Maximum likelihood fitting of general risk models to stratified data. *Appl. Stat.*, **32**, 177–181 (1983).
40. Thomas, D. C. General relative risk models for survival time and matched case-control analysis. *Biometrics*, **37**, 673–686 (1981).
41. Thomas, D. C. Temporal effects and interactions in cancer: Implications of carcinogenic models. *In* "Environmental Health: Risk Assessment," ed. R. L. Prentice and A. S. Whittemore, pp. 107–121 (1982). SIAM, Philadelphia.
42. Tokunaga, M., Land, C. E., Yamamoto, T., Asano, M., Tokuoka, S., Ezaki, H., and Nishimori, I. Incidence of female breast cancer among atomic bomb survivors, Hiroshima and Nagasaki, 1950–80. RERF Tech. Rep. 15-84 (1984).
43. Wakabayashi, T., Kato, H., Ideda, T., and Schull, W. J. Studies of the mortality of A-bomb survivors, Report 7. Part III. Incidence of cancer in 1959–78, based on the Tumor Registry data, Nagasaki. *Radiat. Res.*, **93**, 112–146 (1983).
44. Woolson, W. A., Gritzner, M. L., and Egbert, S. D. Atomic bomb survivor dosimetry. Report to RERF, Dec. 1984.
45. Yamada, Y., Land, C. E., and Hayakawa, N. Interaction between radiation dose and host factors. An epidemiological case-control study of female breast cancer in atomic bomb survivors. RERF Res. Protoc. 14-79 (1979).
46. Yamamoto, T., Moriyama, I. M., Asano, M., and Guralnick, L. The Autopsy Program and the Life Span Study, January 1961–December 1975. RERF Tech. Rep. 18-78 (1978).

EXPERIMENTAL RADIATION CARCINOGENESIS IN RODENTS

Kenjiro YOKORO, Toshio SEYAMA, and Kazuyoshi YANAGIHARA
*Department of Pathology, Research Institute for Nuclear Medicine and Biology, Hiroshima University**

Leukemia, lymphoma, and mammary tumors induced in rodents by ionizing radiation appear, in many aspects, to be the counterparts to those in man as have been observed among the atomic-bomb (A-bomb) survivors.

The emphasis of radiation-induced leukemogenesis was placed on the induction of lymphoid leukemia originating in the thymus (thymic lymphoma), which is most frequently encountered in irradiated mice. In addition to the well-defined factors governing the development and progression of the disease, recent developing interest on the etiological implication of retroviruses and cellular oncogenes is also discussed.

Radiation-induced mammary carcinogenesis in rats is a suitable model for study of human breast cancer with regard to their hormone responsiveness. Our experimental observations using various radiations with different energies in combination with prolactin are described, emphasizing the key role of the promotion phase in carcinogenesis. The experimental system enabled us to demonstrate a high relative biological effectiveness (RBE) of fission spectrum neutrons, which may indicate strong contribution of fission neutrons in induction of malignant tumors among survivors.

The principal late effect of ionizing radiation is the development of cancer in various tissues of man and animals. Among these, leukemia-lymphoma and mammary tumors are most frequently encountered in certain species including man as evidenced by observations in atomic bomb (A-bomb) survivors. In this report, therefore, the description will be limited to these two neoplasms induced in experimental animals by exposure to ionizing radiation; leukemia-lymphoma in mice is reviewed at some length, giving emphasis to the induction mechanism, and mammary tumors in rats in a brief manner calling attention to the high relative biological effectiveness of fission spectrum neutrons.

I. RADIATION-INDUCED LEUKEMOGENESIS IN MICE

Introduction and Historical Background

Leukemia is one of the best known neoplasms causally related to radiation exposure both in man and animals. The first report by Van Jagic *et al.* (*128*) on the leukemogenic effect of radiation in man has been amply confirmed by many investigators (*24*, *97*, *123*). These early findings in man and data accumulated for experimental animals enabled

* Kasumi 1-2-3, Minami-ku, Hiroshima 734, Japan (横路謙次郎, 瀬山敏雄, 柳原五吉).

experts to predict that an excess incidence of leukemia and other neoplasms would occur among survivors exposed to atomic radiation in Hiroshima and Nagasaki (*1*).

Although experimental studies on radiation-induced leukemogenesis have been pursued in several animal species, studies in mice have been most fruitful in producing many valuable insights into leukemogenesis. This review will deal, then, with radiogenic leukemia in mice. The leukemogenic effect of ionizing radiation in mice was first demonstrated in the early 1930s independently by Krebs *et al.* (*80*), Hueper (*49*), and Furth and Furth (*22*). These investigators observed the development of various types of leukemia in X-irradiated mice with a several-fold increased incidence compared to that in non-irradiated controls. Among these pioneers, Furth and Furth (*22*) described not only the induction of leukemia, but also that of other solid neoplastic lesions in three different irradiated mouse strains, thus demonstrating the powerful tumorigenic potency of ionizing radiation.

In the meantime, Furth (*19*) and Furth *et al.* (25) succeeded in establishing a mouse strain, Ak (presently known as AKR) in which lymphoma or lymphoid leukemia, originating mainly in the thymus, occurs spontaneously at a high rate before reaching one year of age. The viral nature of Ak leukemia was later shown by Gross (*27*, *28*) who isolated a leukemogenic type-C RNA virus from leukemic tissue (passage A virus of Gross).

The leukemogenic potency of certain chemicals (*8*, *23*) and of estrogenic hormones (*82*) in mice was also demonstrated in the 1930s. Thus, such agents as radiation, chemicals, hormones, and virus, presently recognized as leukemogens had already been discovered more than four decades ago.

The epoch-making discoveries in leukemia research are as follows:

1. Recognition of leukemogenic potency of radiation, chemicals, and hormones. Furth and Furth (1936), Krebs *et al.* (1930), Hueper (1934), Burrows and Cook (1936), Furth and Furth (1938), Lacassagne (1937).
2. Creation of a high leukemic mouse strain, Ak (AKR), and isolation of a leukemogenic virus from Ak lymphoma. Furth *et al.* (1933), Gross (1951).
3. Demonstration of "indirect induction mechanism" in radiation leukemogenesis, and isolation of a leukemogenic virus (Radiation Leukemia Virus, Rad LV) from radiation-induced lymphoma of C57BL/Ka mice. Kaplan *et al.* (1956), Lieberman and Kaplan (1959).
4. Isolation of leukemogenic viruses from transplantable, solid mouse tumors, such as Friend, Graffi, Moloney, and Rauscher viruses.
5. Proposal of "oncogene hypothesis"; concept of endogenous RNA viruses, and their role in leukemogenesis. Huebner and Todaro (1969).
6. Role of recombinant virus (mink cell focus-inducing, MCF virus) in leukemogenesis; mode of its involvement Hartley *et al.* (1977), Lee and Ihle (1979), Hayward *et al.* (1981), Fischinger *et al.* (1982), Tress *et al.* (1982), Rassart *et al.* (1983).

Type of Leukemia

1. Thymic lymphoma (localized and generalized)

This type of lymphoma (leukemia), originating in the thymus, is far more frequently encountered than the other types of leukemia in many common mouse strains following exposure to ionizing radiation. A high incidence of thymic lymphoma with a short latent period can be obtained by appropriately fractionated whole-body irradiation rather than with a single dose (*69*). A detailed histological study (*115*) revealed that the disease may be initiated unilaterally in an atrophic lobe, followed by invasion into the other lobe, and later forming a huge tumor mass occupying the thoracic cavity. The localized lymphoma eventually disseminates into the visceral organs and the peripheral blood becomes leukemic, the form of which may be the counterpart of acute lymphoid leukemia in children. The tumor cells are morphologically lymphoblastic and carry a cell surface antigen (Thy. 1) which is specific for the T lymphocyte.

2. *Granulocytic (myeloid) leukemia*

Myeloid leukemia in mice, developing either spontaneously or induced by leukemogenic agents, is much less commonly encountered and has been less extensively studied than lymphoid leukemia. The RF (RFM, RF/Jax) strain of mice, originally developed by Furth (*19*) as a low leukemic strain, is a remarkable exception. Upton *et al.* (*124–126*) and Hiraki *et al.* (*44*) reported that myeloid leukemia developed in as high as 40%–50% of young adult male RF mice following a single exposure to 150–450 rad of X-rays. However, in a later study, a much lower incidence of myeloid leukemia was reported in irradiated RF mice maintained under a special pathogen-free condition (*122*). The latent period was slightly longer than that of thymic lymphoma; a majority of cases appeared between 5 to 18 months after irradiation. Myeloid leukemia is characterized by the development of prominent splenomegaly and the appearance of immature granulocytic cells in the peripheral blood. The thymus is usually atrophic. In some cases, leukemic tissue exhibits a yellowish-green color, which is considered to be the counterpart of chloroma or chloroleukemia in man. The disease should be distinguished from leukemoid reaction which is accompanied by infections or amyloidosis.

3. *Nonthymic lymphoma and reticulum cell sarcoma*

These tumors occur much later in life than other types of leukemias. The influence of radiation in induction of nonthymic lymphoma has not been clearly demonstrated, although an increased incidence has been observed in thymectomized mice following exposure to single whole-body irradiation (*124*). RF mice exposed to a single dose of irradiation, either gamma rays or neutrons, show a decrease in the incidence of reticulum cell sarcoma (*122*).

Stemming from the mouse system, modern lymphocytology now contributes much to the progress of fundamental and clinical medicine. The present classification of mouse leukemia is based mainly on the morphology of leukemic cells. A new classification based not only the morphological but also immunological characteristics should be introduced as has been attempted in the human system.

Factors Influencing Radiation-induced Leukemogenesis

It has been well documented that the induction pattern of radiogenic leukemia is modified to a large extent by radiological, physiological, and environmental factors. Kaplan and his associates at Stanford University, who used C57BL/Ka mice as the model system, have made many contributions to the fundamental knowledge of radiogenic thymic lymphoma (*63*, *65*). Studies conducted on RF mice by Upton (*124*) and currently by Ullrich *et al.* (*121*) have furnished a great deal of information on myeloid leukemia.

isolation of a lymphomagenic virus, the Rad LV, which led them to conclude that Rad LV is the direct etiological agent of radiation-induced lymphomas of this mouse strain.

Their interpretation was supported by the electron microscopic demonstration of type-C virus particles in the lymphoreticular tissue of mice shortly after receiving the leukemogenic dose of whole-body X-irradiation (*30*) and by the demonstration of leukemogenic activity of centrifugates derived from the thymus and bone marrow of X-irradiated nonleukemic mice (*34*). These findings were strengthened by similar observations of others in the next few years (*45, 52, 56, 84*). The demonstration that chemically- or hormonally-induced mouse lymphomas (*3, 53, 81, 119*) were transmissible by cell-free extracts gave additional support to the belief that these leukemogenic agents acted merely as the trigger for the activation of a latent leukemogenic virus already present in the host. However, the origins, mode of transmission, and site or mode of residence of the proposed virus were left unknown.

2. *Oncogene hypothesis and endogenous RNA viruses*

In 1969, Huebner and Todaro (*48*) proposed the hypothesis that genetic information for producing C-type RNA viruses is preserved in every vertebra cell and is vertically transmitted from parent to offspring, and this viral information (virogene including oncogene) plays a key role in transforming a normal cell to a tumor cell. According to the hypothesis, tumorigenic treatment and normal aging trigger the activation of endogenous viral information.

The genetically transmitted endogenous RNA viruses have been subdivided into three classes according to their host range: ecotropic, xenotropic, and amphotropic. The MCF virus, a recombinant virus of ecotropic and xenotropic viruses with amphotropic host range is suspected to be most proximately involved in the development of spontaneous lymphomas (*11, 26, 39*).

The oncogene hypothesis had considerable impact upon attempts to understand the mechanism of oncogenesis, and its feasibility has been tested in a variety of experimental systems.

Kaplan (*64*) deduced that at least four different effects of ionizing radiation, acting almost simultaneously in the irradiated host, each contribute to the development of lymphoma following whole-body irradiation: 1) activation of endogenous MuLV replication and mobilization of the virus to the thymus, 2) injury to the thymus followed by a vigorous regeneration, 3) injury to the bone marrow, which in turn interferes with a smooth regeneration of the injured thymus, leading to a state of maturation arrest in which a large number of immature T-lymphocytes become available to interact with the mobilized virus for a sufficient period of time, and 4) immunosuppression caused by both irradiation and MuLV infection, possibly facilitating the proliferation of incipient tumor cells which might have acquired a new antigenic property. An observation of Yokoro *et al.* (*138*) that young adult rats which are otherwise resistant to lymphoma induction by the Gross MuLV could be made susceptible to the virus by a sublethal preirradiation of the rats seems to agree with Kaplan's interpretation.

Nagao (*105*) investigated the appearance of ecotropic MuLV infectivity in various tissues of intact, partial-body shielded or thymectomized female ICR/JCL mice following leukemogenic fractionated X-irradiation to evaluate the correlation between endogenous MuLV infectivity and development of lymphoma in each group. The results indicate that the expression of MuLV may not necessarily be related to the development of lymphoma. Decleve *et al.* (*13*) studied the appearance of Rad LV-associated antigen-positive cells in tissues of C57BL/Ka mice following inoculation of Rad LV which was thought to be the causative agent of radiogenic lymphomas in C57BL/Ka mice. They demonstrated that antigen-positive cells emerged only in the thymus but never in other tissues, the number of positive cells in the thymus increasing gradually during the incubation period, and eventually leading to development of thymic lymphoma. A similar observation was made in W/Fu rats inoculated at birth with the Gross MuLV, in which the exclusive replication of infectious virus in the thymus was associated with the development of thymic lymphomas (*77*).

In contrast to the above, Rad LV-associated antigen-positive cells were rarely found in any tissues of C57BL/Ka mice following leukemogenic X-irradiation (*91*). Ihle *et al.* (*50*, *51*) demonstrated in C57BL/6 mice that, although the expression of endogenous ecotropic MuLV was accelerated by leukemogenic irradiation, the peak titer of antibody against gp 71 of the endogenous ecotropic MuLV in irradiated mice was comparable to that in nonirradiated controls, and that the antibody titers were never affected by procedures which lower the leukemia incidence, such as irradiating older mice, low dose irradiation and postirradiation bone marrow transplantation. Furthermore, with rare exceptions, expression of viral antigens was not detected in induced lymphomas. These and other findings (*98*) indicate that the endogenous viruses, at least of ecotropic MuLV, are not playing a major role in mouse radiation-induced leukemogenesis. Moreover, the etiological role of ecotropic MuLV has been negated in chemically-induced leukemogenesis (*106*, *107*).

On the other hand, the transient appearance of MuLV gs antigen-positive cells in the bone marrow and thymus of mice several weeks after X-irradiation was interpreted as evidence for the viral involvement even though there was no viral expression in the established lymphoma cells (*33*). Rassart *et al.* (*111*) and Sankar-Mistry *et al.* (*113*) reported that the recombinant B-tropic virus with ecotropic host range is regularly released from cell lines derived from radiogenic lymphomas in C57BL/Ka mice, emphasizing the etiological role of the virus in radiogenic leukemogenesis. However, our observation that there is no evidence of viral implication in cell lines established from radiation- or chemically-induced lymphomas in NFS/N mice may still raise a question to their notion (*136*). There is a report (*92*) suggesting an inhibitory effect of interferon in radiation- and Rad LV-induced leukemogenesis when the leukemogenic stimuli were submaximal. On the contrary, our recent observations that radiation- and chemically-induced mouse leukemogenesis was not affected by treatment with beta-type mouse interferon, while leukemia induction with the Gross MuLV was completely inhibited by the same treatment, also appear to favor the nonviral mechanism of radiation leukemogenesis (Yokoro *et al.* unpublished data).

3. *Recently proposed hypothesis*

Although MCF virus is the likely etiologic agent in leukemic strains such as AKR and C58 mice, there are no reports suggesting direct involvement of infectious MCF virus in radiation-induced leukemogenesis in low leukemic strains. If so, how are endogenous MuLVs implicated and what is the likely mechanism of radiation-induced leukemogenesis? The following are the hypotheses recently proposed by some investigators.

A) *Virus promoter insertion hypothesis*

This was first proposed by Hayward *et al.* (*42*) in induction of B-cell lymphoma by avian leukosis virus which is devoid of viral oncogene (v-onc). They stated that development of lymphoma is due to the activation of a cellular oncogene (c-onc) through the insertion of a viral promoter sequence adjacent to the c-onc. Repeated virus infection might be required for the insertion of the promoter at an appropriate location, which may account for a long latent period of MuLV-induced leukemogenesis as compared to that of sarcoma induction by murine sarcoma virus (MuSV) that possesses v-onc. Observations in murine virus-induced lymphomas suggest that lymphomagenesis by MuLVs can result from insertional mutagenesis of cellular oncogenes (*116*).

B) *Receptor-mediated leukemogenesis*

McGrath and Weissmann (*100*, *101*) proposed the receptor-mediated leukemogenesis hypothesis in which the continued presentation of MuLV env determinant to the cell surface receptor would act as mitogenic stimuli for the replication of MuLV-induced lymphoma cells. Ellis *et al.* (*15*) and Tress *et al.* (120) stated that leukemogenesis does not show a simple dependence on infectious MuLV expression in radiogenic lymphomas, and that the expression of recombinant env gene product on the lymphoma cells might play an important role in cell replication. A hypothesis along similar lines has also been proposed by Lee and Ihle (*88*). Fischinger *et al.* (*16*), analyzing virus-negative radiogenic lymphoma cells of C57BL/Ka origin, emphasized that binding of nonvirion-associated permuted gp 70s, which are products of radiation-altered proviral DNA, to cell surface receptors might act as the signal for autostimulatory blastogenesis, leading to the selective proliferation of the receptor-bearing T-cells. According to this hypothesis no complete virus infection or expression of other viral antigens would be required.

C) *Oncogene activation*

In the past few years, the association of oncogene activation and lymphomagenesis has been analyzed using both molecular hybridization and gene transfer assays. Activation of the ras gene family appears rather common in the mouse T-cell lymphomas (*32*, *129*). T lym-l gene has been isolated from T-cell lymphoma cell lines by molecular cloning (*83*). In our recent study (*136*), however, there was neither amplification nor rearrangement of env specific genes of MuLV and of cellular oncogenes, such as ras gene family and myc gene in DNA of NFS cell lines derived from radiation- or chemically-induced lymphomas. Nevertheless, a molecular approach to lymphomagenesis should be instrumental in elucidating the induction mechanism.

From these hypotheses and observations, there is no doubt that investigations of viral oncogenesis have contributed much to exploration of the leukemogenic mechanism, in general, and the author feels that the distinction between viral leukemogenesis and that induced by other agents is disappearing.

It may also be inferred that infectious endogenous MuLVs as the main cause of radiation-induced leukemogenesis is probably a rare event, if it occurs at all, but may rather play a role in certain processes in ways different from those hitherto conceived. The occasional isolation of leukemogenic viruses from radiation-induced lymphomas may well represent a rare event.

II. RADIATION-INDUCED MAMMARY CARCINOGENESIS IN RATS

There have been many reports dealing with the mammary carcinogenic effect of large doses of low LET radiation in rats (*13*, *14*, *16*), while that of high LET radiation in low dose ranges has yet to be adequately evaluated. In this review, we present the relevant data in rats recently obtained in our laboratory (*27*, *28*).

Mammary Carcinogenic Effect of Low Dose Fission Neutrons and Other Radiations

1. *Induction of mammary tumor (MT) with low doses of fission spectrum neutrons*

Studies were undertaken to evaluate the carcinogenic effect of fission neutrons in the low dose range, and the results were compared with those obtained from experiments with 180 kilovolt peak (KvP) X-rays, 14.1 MeV fast neutrons, and 0–0 25 eV thermal neutrons. The rat mammary tumor system has the following advantage as an experimental model for human breast cancer; 1) rat MT is readily induced either by radiation or chemical carcinogens, 2) many rats MTs are hormone dependent or hormone responsive, 3) the majority of rat MTs are of ductal origin as is the case in human, and 4) an increased risk of breast cancer has been observed among women exposed to A-bomb radiation (*19–21*).

Female W/Fu rats were irradiated at 50 days of age at the Research Reactor Institute, Kyoto University. Irradiation field equivalent to the Hiroshima A-bomb was realized by use of a fission plate (uranium energy converter) Thermal neutrons with an energy of 0.025 eV from the heavy-water thermal neutron facility of KUR (5 mW) (*5*) at a neutron flux of 3×10^{9} n/cm^{2}/sec hit the fission plate; then fast neutrons with average energy of 2.0 MeV and prompt gamma rays were produced by fission reaction of ^{235}U. About 50% of the radiation-initiated rats were further treated with prolactin, the physiological regulatory hormone of mammary tissue, as a promoter to facilitate the detection of the

TABLE I. Induction of MT in Female W/Fu Rats by a Combined Treatment of Fission Radiation and Prolactin

Treatment	Rat with MT / Number in group	Number of MT	Type of MT: Adenoca.	Type of MT: Fibroad.	Latency of MT after irradiation (days)
None	2/24 (8.3%)	3	0	3	597, 843
Prolactin	0/14	—	—	—	—
1.1 rad alone[a]	1/14 (7.1)	1	1	—	304
4.1 rad alone[b]	1/16 (6.3)	1	—	1	205
7.3 rad alone[c]	0/16	—	—	—	—
16.6 rad alone[d]	0/16	—	—	—	—
1.1 rad+prolactin[e]	1/15 (6.7)	1	1	—	237
4.1 rad+prolactin	6/16 (37.5)	6	5	1	191–334
7.3 rad+prolactin	5/15 (33.3)	5	3	2	165–365
16.6 rad+prolactin	9/17 (52.9)	13	7	6	163–365
1.1 rad+prolactin[f]	1/6 (16.7)	1	1	—	502
4.1 rad+prolactin	4/15 (26.7)	6	5	1	463–567
7.3 rad+prolactin	3/15 (20.0)	5	4	1	504–549
16.6 rad+prolactin	4/15 (26.7)	6	5	1	375–526

[a] 0.3 rad fission neutron+0.8 rad gamma rays.
[b] 1.7 rad fission neutron+2.4 rad gamma rays.
[c] 3.3 rad fission neutron+4.0 rad gamma rays.
[d] 8.1 rad fission neutron+8.5 rad gamma rays.
[e] Supply of prolactin was started shortly after irradiation.
[f] Supply of prolactin was started 12 months after irradiation.

carcinogenic effect of radiation. Prolactin was started either a few days or 12 months after irradiation. Experiments were terminated 12–18 months after irradiation.

The incidence, histological type, and latency period of MT in rats of various groups are summarized in Table I. Only 2 of 62 (3.2%) rats receiving 1.0, 4.1, 7.3, or 16.6 rad of fission radiation (composed of both 2.0 MeV fission spectrum neutrons and gamma rays) alone developed MT of benign fibroadenoma type with a long latency period. The induction rate was similar to that of nonirradiated controls. In contrast, 21 of 63 (33.3%) irradiated rats developed MT with a short latency if prolactin was started shortly after irradiation as shown in the middle rows of Table I. The majority of induced MTs were malignant adenocarcinomas. Of 16 rats 6 (37.5%) had MT following exposure to 4.1 rad of fission radiation which contained only 1.7 rad of fission neutron component. The long survival of radiation-initiated potentially malignant cells was apparent when the supply of prolactin to irradiated rats was delayed as late as 12 months after irradiation; 12 of 51 (23.7%) rats developed MT, the frequency of which was comparable to that in rats given prolactin shortly after irradiation (Table I). It is interesting to note that the relative efficacy of MT induction by low dose range of fission radiation appears to be dose independent, the lower dose produced a higher relative risk.

The growth of adenocarcinomas induced by combined treatment of radiation and prolactin was shown to be dependent on both prolactin and ovarian hormones as demonstrated by growth retardation and shrinkage of MT following resection of either grafted prolactin-secreting pituitary tumor or oophorectomy, or both.

2. *MT inductivity of ^{60}Co gamma rays in low dose range*

The mammary carcinogenic effect of gamma rays was tested in order to evaluate the role of gamma rays, which is one component of fission radiation. None of 40 rats exposed to 10 rad of ^{60}Co gamma rays with or without prolactin supply developed MT in an observation period of 12 months, indicating that fission spectrum neutrons played a major role in induction of MT in combination with prolactin.

3. *Relative Biological Effectiveness (RBE) of fission spectrum neutrons in induction of rat MT*

As stated above, fission spectrum neutrons, especially in the low dose range, were shown to be highly carcinogenic on rat mammary tissue. Therefore, RBE of fission spectrum neutrons for the rat MT inductivity was compared with that of 180 KvP X-rays, 14.1 MeV fast neutrons (*27*, *28*) and 0.025 eV thermal neutrons (unpublished data). We estimated the RBE in such a way as to compare the dose of each radiation type that would produce a MT frequency which was 40% of the incidence in irradiated rats treated with prolactin. The doses of each radiation type which induced 40% incidence were: 50 rad of X-rays, 35.4 rad of fast neutrons, 7.4 rad of thermal neutrons, and 2.8 rad

TABLE II. Differences in MT Inductivity of Various Radiations in Female W/Fu Rats as Detected by the Promotive Effect of Prolactin

	Fission neutrons (2.0 MeV)	Thermal neutrons (0.025 eV)	Fast neutrons (14.1 MeV)	X-rays (180 kVp)
Dose (rad) giving 40% of MT incidence	2.8	7.4	35.4	50
RBE for MT inductivity	17.8	6.7	1.4	1

of fission neutrons, respectively. Since gamma rays play a minor role in rat mammary carcinogenesis as described in the previous section, the gamma ray component was arbitrarily ignored for the latter two radiation types. As shown in Table II, it is clear that the efficiency of 2.0 MeV fission spectrum neutrons is much higher than those of others; RBE of fission spectrum neutrons is 17.8 against 180 KvP X-rays.

DISCUSSION

We have demonstrated that the mammary carcinogenic effect of apparently sub-carcinogenic doses of fission neutrons could be promoted by elevating prolactin levels in irradiated rats.

The determining role of prolactin in the induction and maintenance of the growth of murine mammary carcinogenesis has been well documented (*3*, *6*, *9*, *18*, *24–26*), from which the importance of prolactin in human breast carcinogenesis is easily conceived. However, the findings have been conflicting with respect to the serum prolactin levels of breast cancer patients (*1*, *4*, *8*, *12*, *17*). Taking a general view of the implication of prolactin in normal and transformed mammary epithelial cells in both rodents and humans, it is assumed that the elevation of prolactin level to a certain extent, with other favorable host factors, is a prerequisite for the induction and further development of MT regardless of the species.

It has been well documented that the relative risk of MT has been increasing among women who were exposed to A-bomb radiation, and the effect is dose dependent (*19–21*). The long latency of MT development among survivors suggests that long-surviving radiation-initiated dormant cancer cells may exist in the mammary tissue and that those cancer cells begin to proliferate in response to the change in certain host and other environmental factors. This supposition is supported by our data in rats (*27*, *28*).

Vogel (*22*), Vogel and Zaldiver (*23*), and Shellabarger *et al.* (*15*) reported an extremely high RBE of 0.43 MeV or 1.2 MeV fission neutrons as compared with 250 KvP X-rays for the induction of rat MT. Montour *et al.* (*7*) and Clifton *et al.* (*2*) also stressed the high efficiency of neutrons in different experimental systems. Furthermore, all these authors emphasized that the high RBE of neutrons was more prominent in the low dose range and that the RBE of neutrons decreases as dose increases.

CLOSING REMARKS

Almost half a century has passed since experimental study, mainly of mice, was introduced as a model system for studying the etiology, pathophysiology, and treatment of human leukemia. At present, a counterpart for almost every form of human leukemia can be induced in rodents by the skillful use of various leukemogens including ionizing radiation. Furthermore, recent advances in immunology, genetics, tumor virology, and molecular biology have been incorporated into leukemia research, resulting in rapid progress, especially with respect to T-cell lymphoma and lymphoid leukemia.

Continued efforts along these lines will enable us to arrive at a unified concept of radiation-induced leukemogenesis in the not too distant future.

The experimental findings described in this review, particularly those related to radiation-induced mammary carcinogenesis, may have some relevance to the recent investigations for reassessment of gamma ray and neutron radiation dose produced by the A-bombs in Hiroshima and Nagasaki (*10*, *11*). Although our evidence shows that neutrons can be effective in animal carcinogenesis, there seems no human population available for comparison, since it is now known that the neutron dose in Hiroshima and Nagasaki was so small that the effects cannot be adequately assessed.

Acknowledgment

All of our studies described in this review were performed under the support of a Grant-in-Aid for Cancer Research from the Ministry of Education, Science and Culture, Japan.

REFERENCES

I. Radiation-Induced Leukemogenesis in Mice

1. A review of thirty years study of Hiroshima and Nagasaki atomic bomb survivors, *J. Radiat. Res.*, **16** (Suppl.), 1–164 (1975).
2. Azumi, J. and Sachs, L. Chromosome mapping of the genes that control differentiation and malignancy in myeloid leukemia cells. *Proc. Natl. Acad. Sci. U.S.A.*, **74**, 253–257 (1977).
3. Ball, J. K. and McCarter, J. A. Repeated demonstration of a mouse leukemia virus after treatment with chemical carcinogens. *J. Natl. Cancer Inst.*, **46**, 751–762 (1971).
4. Bessho, M. and Hirashima, K. Experimental studies on the mechanism of leukemogenesis following the hemopoietic stem cell kinetics. *Acta Haematol. Jpn.*, **45**, 1296–1306 (1982).
5. Boniver, J., Decleve, A., Lieberman, M., Honsik, C., Travis, M., and Kaplan, H. S. Marrow-thymus interactions during radiation leukemogenesis in C57BL/Ka mice. *Cancer Res.*, **41**, 390–392 (1981).
6. Boniver, J., Simar, L. J., Courtoy, R., and Betz, E. H. Quantitative analysis of thymus lymphoid cells during murine radioleukemogenesis. *Cancer Res.*, **38**, 52–58 (1978).
7. Brues, A. M., Aacher, G. A., Finkel, M. P., and Lisco, H. Comparative carcinogenic effects by X-radiation and P^{32}. *Cancer Res.*, **9**, 545 (1949).
8. Burrows, H. and Cook, J. W. Spindle-cell tumours and leucaemia in mice after injection with a water soluble compound of 1:2:5:6-dibenzanthracene. *Am J. Cancer*, **27**, 267–278 (1936).
9. Carnes, W. H., Kaplan, H. S., Brown, M. B., and Hirsch, B. B. Indirect induction of lymphomas in irradiated mice. III. Role of the thymic graft. *Cancer Res.*, **16**, 429–433 (1956).
10. Chan, F.P.H., Ball, J. K., and Sergovich, F. R. Trisomy #15 in murine thymomas induced by chemical carcinogens, x-irradiation, and an endogenous murine leukemia virus. *J. Natl. Cancer Inst.*, **62**, 605–610 (1979).
11. Cloyd, M. W., Hartley, J. W., and Rowe, W. P. Lymphomagenicity of recombinant mink cell focus-inducing murine leukemia viruses. *J. Exp. Med.*, **151**, 542–552 (1980).
12. Congdon, C. C., Uphoff, D., and Lorenz, E. Modification of acute irradiation injury in mice and guinea pigs by injection of bone marrow: A histopathologic study. *J. Natl. Cancer Inst.*, **13**, 73–107 (1952).
13. Decleve, A., Sato, C., Lieberman, M., and Kaplan, H. S. Selective thymic localization of murine leukemia virus-related antigens in C57BL/Ka mice after inoculation with Radiation Leukemia Virus. *Proc. Natl. Acad. Sci. U.S.A.*, **71**, 3124–3128 (1974).
14. Dofuku, R., Biedler, J. L., Spengler, B. A., and Old, L. J. Trisomy of chromosome 15 in spontaneous leukemias of AKR mice. *Proc. Natl. Acad. Sci. U.S.A.*, **72**, 1515–1517 (1975).
15. Ellis, R. W., Stockert, E., and Fleissner, E. Association of endogenous retroviruses with radiation-induced leukemias of BALB/c mice. *J. Virol.*, **33**, 652–660 (1980).

16. Fischinger, P. J., Thiel, H. J., Lieberman, M., Kaplan, H. S., Dunlop, N. M. and Robey, W. G. Presence of a novel recombinant murine leukemia virus-like glycoprotein on the surface of virus-negative C57BL lymphoma cells. *Cancer Res.*, **42**, 4650–4657 (1982).
17. Ford, C. E., Hamerton, J. L., and Mole, R. H. Chromosomal changes in primary and transplanted reticular neoplasms of the mouse. *J. Cell Comp. Physiol.*, **1** (Suppl.), 235–269 (1958).
18. Fry, R.J.M., Experimental radiation carcinogenesis: What have we learned? *Radiat. Res.*, **87**, 224–239 (1981).
19. Furth, J. The creation of the AKR strain, whose DNA contains the genome of a leukemia virus. *In* "Origins of Inbred Mice," ed. H. C. Morse III, pp. 69–97 (1978). Academic Press, New York.
20. Furth, J. and Boon, M. C. Enhancement of leukemogenic action of methylcholanthrene by preirradiation with x-rays. *Science*, **98**, 133–139 (1943).
21. Furth, J. and Boon, M. C. The time and site of origin of the leukemic cells. AAAS Research Conference on Cancer, pp. 129–138 (1944).
22. Furth, J. and Furth, O. B. Neoplastic disease produced in mice by general irradiation with x-rays. 1. Incidence and type of neoplasms. *Am. J. Cancer*, **28**, 54–65 (1936).
23. Furth, J. and Furth, O. B. Monocytic leukemia and other neoplastic diseases occurring in mice following intrasplenic injection of 1: 2-benzpyrene. *Am. J. Cancer*, **34**, 169–183 (1938).
24. Furth, J. and Lorenz, E. Carcinogenesis by ionizing radiation. *In* "Radiation Biology," ed. A. Hollander, pp. 1145–1201 (1954). McGraw Hill, New York.
25. Furth, J., Seibold, H. R., and Rathbone, R. R. Experimental studies on lymphomatosis of mice. *Am. J. Cancer*, **19**, 521–604 (1933).
26. Green, N., Hiai, H., Elder, J. H., Schwartz, R. S., Khiroya, R. H., Thomas, C. Y., Tsichles, P. N., and Coffin, J. M. Expression of leukemogenic recombinant viruses associated with a recessive gene in HRS/J mice. *J. Exp. Med.*, **152**, 249–264 (1980).
27. Gross, L. "Spontaneous" leukemia developing in C3H mice following inoculation, in infancy, with Ak-leukemic extracts, or Ak-embryos. *Proc. Soc. Exp. Biol. Med.*, **76**, 27–32 (1951).
28. Gross, L. Development and serial cell-free passage of a highly potent strain of mouse leukemia virus. *Proc. Soc. Exp. Biol. Med.*, **94**, 767–771 (1957).
29. Gross, L. Serial cell-free passage of a radiation-activated mouse leukemia agent. *Proc. Soc. Exp. Biol. Med.*, **100**, 102–105 (1959).
30. Gross, L. and Feldman, G. G. Electron microscopic studies of radiation-induced leukemia in mice: virus release following total-body x-ray irradiation. *Cancer Res.*, **28**, 1677–1685 (1968).
31. Gross, L., Roswit, B., Mada, E. R., Dreyfuss, Y., and Moore, L. A. Studies on radiation-induced leukemia in mice. *Cancer Res.*, **19**, 316–320 (1959).
32. Guerrero, I., Calzada, P., Mayer, A., and Pellicer, A. A molecular approach to leukemogenesis: Mouse lymphomas contain an activated c-ras oncogene. *Proc. Natl. Acad. Sci. U.S.A.*, **81**, 202–205 (1984).
33. Haas, M. Transient virus expression during murine leukemia induction by x-irradiation. *J. Natl. Cancer Inst.*, **58**, 251–257 (1977).
34. Haran-Ghera, N. Leukemogenic activity of centrifugates from irradiated mouse thymus and bone marrow. *Int. J. Cancer*, **1**, 81–87 (1966).
35. Haran-Ghera, N. Pathways in murine radiation leukemogenesis-coleukemogenesis. *In* "Biology of Radiation Carcinogenesis," ed. J. Yuhas, R. Tennant, and J. Regen, pp. 245–260 (1976). Raven Press, New York.
36. Haran-Ghera, N. Target cells involved in radiation leukemia virus leukemogenesis. *In*

"International Symposium on Radiation Induced Leukemogenesis and Related Viruses, INSERM Symp. No. 4," ed. J. F. Duplan, pp. 79–89 (1977). Elsevier/North Holland Biomedical Press, Amsterdam.

37. Haran-Ghera, N. and Kaplan, H. S. Significance of thymus and marrow injury in urethan leukemogenesis. *Cancer Res.*, **24**, 1926–1931 (1964).
38. Haran-Ghera, N. and Peled, A. The mechanism of radiation action in leukemogenesis. IV. Immune impairment as a coleukemogenic factor. *Isr. J. Med. Sci.*, **4**, 1181–1187 (1968).
39. Hartley, J. W., Wolford, N. K., Old, L. J., and Rowe, W. P. A new class of murine leukemia virus associated with development of spontaneous lymphomas. *Proc. Natl. Acad. Sci. U.S.A.*, **74**, 789–792 (1977).
40. Hayata, I., Ishihara, T., Hirashima, K., Sado, T., and Yamagiwa, J. Partial deletion of chromosome #2 in myelocytic leukemias of irradiated C3H/He and RFM mice. *J. Natl. Cancer Inst.*, **63**, 843–848 (1979).
41. Hayata, I., Seki, M., Yoshida, K., Hirashima, K., Sado, T., Yamagiwa, J., and Ishihara, T. Chromosomal aberrations observed in 52 mouse myeloid leukemias. *Cancer Res.*, **43**, 367–373 (1983).
42. Hayward, W. S., Neel, B. G., and Astrin, S. M. Activation of a cellular onc gene by promoter insertion in ALV-induced lymphoid leukosis. *Nature*, **290**, 475–480 (1981).
43. Hiai, N., Nishi, Y., Miyazawa, T., Matsudaira, Y., and Nishizuka, Y. Mouse lymphoid leukemias: Symbiotic complexes of neoplastic lymphocytes and their microenvironments. *J. Natl. Cancer Inst.*, **66**, 713–722 (1981).
44. Hiraki, K., Irino, S., and Sota, S. Studies on cytogenesis of RF mouse leukemia induced by X-ray irradiation. Proc. 8th Congr. Europ. Soc. Hematol., p. 347 (1962).
45. Hiraki, K., Irino, S., Sota, S., and Ikejiri, K. Leukemogenic activity of cell-free filtrates of radiation-induced leukemia of RF mice. *J. Radiat. Res.*, **5**, 1–11 (1964).
46. Hormberg, E.A.D., De Pasqualini, C. D., Arini, E., Pavlovsky, A., and Rabasa, S. L. Leukemogenic effect of radioactive phosphorous in adult and fetally exposed BALB mice. *Cancer Res.*, **24**, 1745–1748 (1964).
47. Hormberg, E.A.D., Vasquez, C., De Pasqualini, C. D., Pavlovsky, A., and Rabasa, S. L. A cellular passage of ^{32}P-induced leukemia; an electron microscopic study. *Cancer Res.*, **27**, 198–204 (1967).
48. Huebner, R. J. and Todaro, G. J. Oncogenes of RNA tumor viruses as determinants of cancer. *Proc. Natl. Acad. Sci. U.S.A.*, **64**, 1087–1094 (1969).
49. Hueper, W. C. Leukemoid and leukemic conditions in white mice with spontaneous mammary carcinoma. *Folia Haematol.*, **52**, 167–178 (1934).
50. Ihle, J. N., Joseph, D. R., and Pazmino, N. H. Radiation leukemia in C57BL/6 mice. II. Lack of ecotropic virus expression in the majority of lymphomas. *J. Exp. Med.*, **144**, 1406–1423 (1976).
51. Ihle, J. N., McEwan, R., and Bengali, K. Radiation leukemia in C57BL/6 mice. 1. Lack of serological evidence for the role of endogenous ecotropic viruses in pathogenesis. *J. Exp. Med.*, **144**, 1391–1405 (1976).
52. Ilbery, P.L.T. and Winn, S. M. Indirect transfer of radiogenic lymphoma. *Aust. J. Exp. Biol. Med. Sci.*, **42**, 133–148 (1964).
53. Irino, S., Ota, Z., Sezaki, T., Suzaki, M., and Hiraki, K. Cell-free transmission of 20-methylcholanthrene-induced RF mouse leukemia and electron microscopic demonstration of virus particles in its leukemic tissue. *Gann*, **54**, 225–237 (1963).
54. Ito, T., Nagao, K., Kawamura, Y., and Yokoro, K. Studies on the leukemogenic and immunologic effects of radiostrontium (^{90}Sr) and X-rays in mice. *In* "Proc. 14th Annual Hanford Biology Symp. of Radiation and the Lymphatic System, ERDA Symp. Series 37," pp. 209–217 (1976). National Technical Information Service, US Dept. of Commerce, Springfield.

55. Ito, T., Yokoro, K., Ito, A., and Nishihara, E. A comparative study of the leukemogenic effects of strontium-90 and x-rays in mice. *Proc. Soc. Exp. Biol. Med.*, **130**, 345–350 (1969).
56. Jenkins, V. K. and Upton, A. C. Cell-free transmission of radiogenic myeloid leukemia in the mouse. *Cancer Res.*, **23**, 1748–1755 (1963).
57. Joneja, M. G. and Stich, H. F. Chromosomes of tumor cells. IV. Cell population changes in thymus, spleen, and bone marrow during X-ray-induced leukemogenesis in C57BL/6J mice. *J. Natl. Cancer Inst.*, **35**, 421–434 (1965).
58. Kaplan, H. S. Observations on radiation-induced lymphoid tumors of mice. *Cancer Res.*, **7**, 141–147 (1947).
59. Kaplan, H. S. Comparative susceptibility of the lymphoid tissues of strain C57 Black mice to the induction of lymphoid tumors by irradiation. *J. Natl. Cancer Inst.*, **8**, 191–197 (1948).
60. Kaplan, H. S. Preliminary studies on the effectiveness of local irradiation in the induction of lymphoid tumors in mice. *J. Natl. Cancer Inst.*, **10**, 267–270 (1949).
61. Kaplan, H. S. Influence of thymectomy, splenectomy, and gonadectomy on incidence of radiation-induced lymphoid tumors in strain C57 Black mice. *J. Natl. Cancer Inst.*, **11**, 83–90 (1950).
62. Kaplan, H. S. The nature of the neoplastic transformation in lymphoid tumour induction. *In* "Ciba Foundation Symposium on Carcinogenesis, Mechanism of Action," pp. 233–244 (1959). Little Brown, Boston.
63. Kaplan, H. S. On the natural history of the murine leukemias: Presidential address. *Cancer Res.*, **27**, 1325–1340 (1967).
64. Kaplan, H. S. Leukemia and lymphoma in experimental and domestic animals. *Ser. Haemat.*, *VII*, (2), 94–163 (1974).
65. Kaplan, H. S. Interaction between radiation and viruses in the induction of murine thymic lymphomas and lymphatic leukemias. *In* "International Symposium on Radiation-induced Leukemogenesis and Related Viruses, INSERM Symp. No. 4," ed. J. F. Duplan, pp. 1–18 (1977). Elsevier/North Holland Biomedical Press Amsterdam.
66. Kaplan, H. S. and Brown, M. B. Protection against radiation-induced lymphoma development by shielding and partial-body irradiation of mice. *Cancer Res.*, **12**, 441–444 (1952).
67. Kaplan, H. S. and Brown, M. B. Testosterone prevention of post-irradiation lymphomas in C57 Black mice. *Cancer Res.*, **12**, 445–447 (1952).
68. Kaplan, H. S. and Brown, M. B. Mortality of mice after total-body irradiation as influenced by alterations in total dose fractionation, and periodicity of treatment. *J. Natl. Cancer Inst.*, **12**, 765–775 (1952).
69. Kaplan, H. S. and Brown, M. B. A quantitative dose-response study of lymphoid-tumor development in irradiated C57 Black mice. *J. Natl. Cancer Inst.*, **13**, 185–208 (1952).
70. Kaplan, H. S., Brown, M. B., Hirsch, B. B., and Carnes, W. H. Indirect induction of lymphomas in irradiated mice. II. Factor of irradiation of the host. *Cancer Res.*, **16**, 426–428 (1956).
71. Kaplan, H. S., Brown, M. B., and Paull, J. Influence of post-irradiation thymectomy and of thymic implants on lymphoid tumor incidence in C57BL mice. *Cancer Res.*, **13**, 677–680 (1953).
72. Kaplan, H. S., Brown, M. B., and Paull, J. Influence of bone marrow injections on involution and neoplasia of mouse thymus after systemic irradiation. *J. Natl. Cancer. Inst.*, **14**, 303–316 (1953).
73. Kaplan, H. S., Carnes, W. H., Brown, M. B., and Hirsch, B. B. Indirect induction of lymphomas in irradiated mice. 1. Tumor incidence and morphology in mice bearing non-irradiated thymic grafts. *Cancer Res.*, **16**, 422–425 (1956).
74. Kaplan, H. S., Hirsch, B. B., and Brown, M. B. Indirect induction of lymphomas in irradiated mice. IV. Genetic evidence of the origin of the tumor cells from the thymic grafts. *Cancer Res.*, **16**, 434–436 (1956).

was not previously found to be significantly elevated in A-bomb survivors, has gradually increased in heavily exposed persons 20 years after the bomb. Anderson and Ishida (*2*) and Nishiyama *et al.* (*18*) have reported the incidence of malignant lymphoma in A-bomb survivors.

Recently many types of leukemia have been considered stem cell diseases. In A-bomb survivors the incidence of all types of leukemia, except chronic lymphocytic leukemia, has increased and consequently it is suggested that A-bomb radiation initially affected immature hematopoietic stem cells. However, MM is a malignant disease of differentiated B lymphocytes and malignant lymphoma is a disease of mature lymphocytes (usually T- or B-cells) as is chronic lymphocytic leukemia. Thus, the difference in prevalence and period of occurrence of these diseases in A-bomb survivors seems quite interesting in terms of the radiation effect on the hematopoietic system.

In this review, we would like to describe the occurrence and the characteristics of the hematological malignancies among A-bomb survivors and consider the relationship of these diseases to A-bomb radiation.

Estimation of radiation dose for each survivor is important for clarification of the radiation effect. So far, the tentative 1965 dose (T65D) estimates which were estimated in 1965 by Oak Ridge National Laboratory (*17*) have been used for dose estimation of each A-bomb survivor. However, dosimetry of A-bomb radiation in Hiroshima and Nagasaki is now being reassessed after the Lawrence Livermore National Laboratory reported revised A-bomb radiation estimates in 1981 (*15*). This means that the neutron dose in both cities, and especially in Hiroshima, will decrease in the new estimations. As no conclusion has yet been reached, the T65D was used in this review.

A Radiation Effects Research Foundation (RERF) fixed sample of 109,000 subjects (82,000 survivors and 27,000 controls) was used to show the relationship between the incidence of these diseases and A-bomb radiation effects.

Leukemia

Leukemia cases among A-bomb survivors estimated to have received a radiation dose greater than 1 rad increased gradually from 1946 with maximum occurrence ob-

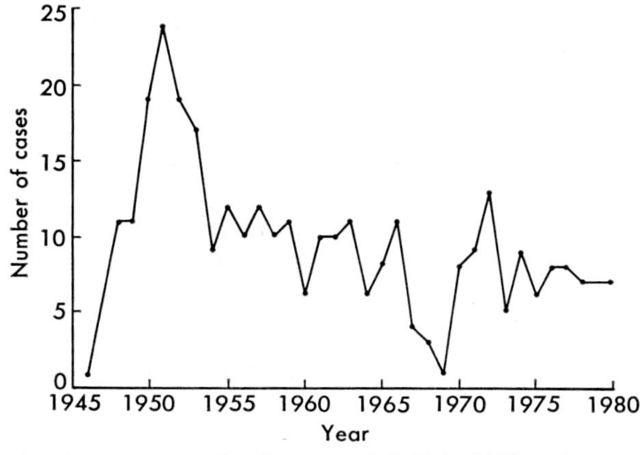

FIG. 1. Leukemia among proximally exposed (within 2000 m from ground zero) A-bomb survivors who received more than 1 rad radiation dose, Hiroshima and Nagasaki, 1945.

served in 1951, six years after the A-bomb. After 1951 the occurrence of leukemia decreased gradually with some fluctuation but there has been no year where the annual incidence among the proximally exposed (within 2,000 m from ground zero) was zero (Fig. 1). We would like to illustrate probable A-bomb induced leukemia using the RERF sample. A total of 189 leukemia cases (149 in Hiroshima and 40 in Nagasaki) have been detected during 1950–78 among these subjects.

Annual Incidence Rate for Leukemia by Dose, City, and Type of Leukemia

Figure 2 shows the crude annual incidence rate in the RERF sample during 1950–78 by dose, city, and two major types of leukemia, acute leukemia and chronic myelogenous leukemia (CML). Note, first, that the risk of all types of leukemia increases with dose in both cities, except for Nagasaki survivors who received less than 100 rad kerma total dose (average marrow total dose). Second, the risk of CML increases among individuals who received less than 50 rad kerma total dose in Hiroshima, but in Nagasaki the risk is significantly increased only among survivors who received 200 rad or more kerma total dose. The shape of the dose-response curves differs between the two cities and for acute leukemia and CML.

Annual Incidence Rate for All Types of Leukemia by Dose, City, Age at Time of Bomb (ATB), and Period

Figure 3 shows the trend of the standardized annual incidence rates for all types of leukemia by dose and city. The excess risk in individuals who received 200 rad or more

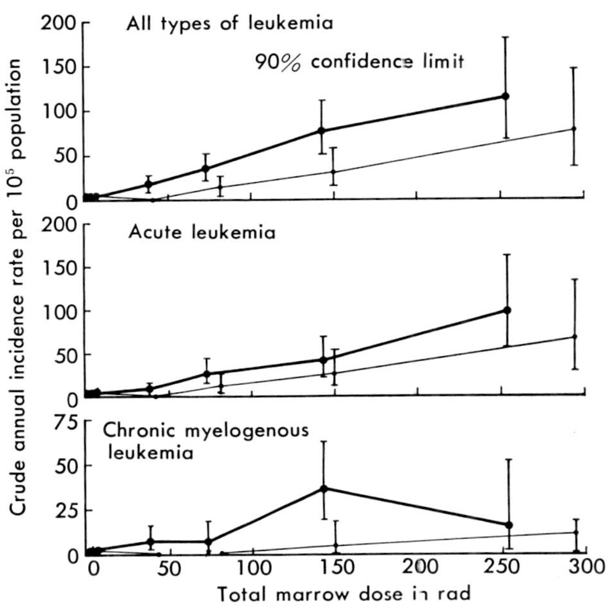

FIG. 2. Crude annual incidence rate for leukemia among A-bomb survivors in the RERF sample by total marrow dose, type of leukemia, and city, 1950–78. ●, Hiroshima; •, Nagasaki.

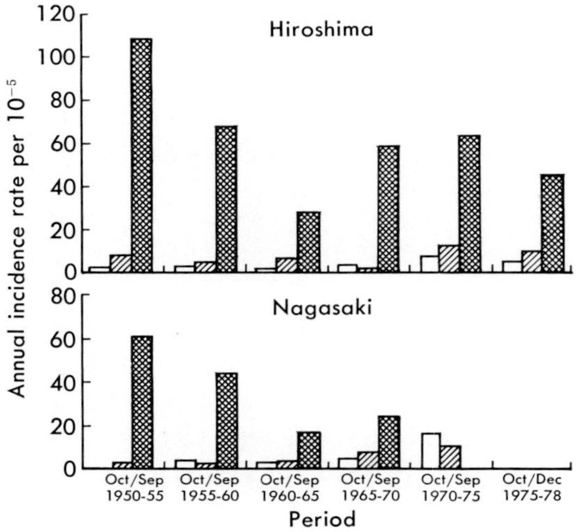

FIG. 3. Standardized annual incidence rate for all types of leukemia in the RERF sample by dose, time period, and city, 1950–78. □, control; ▨, 1–99 rad; ▩, 100+ rad.

kerma total dose has declined with time after exposure in both cities. In Hiroshima the downward trend has been slow and the effect extends to 1978, but in Nagasaki the excess risk declined sharply with time after exposure and disappeared by 1970. Thus, the pattern of disappearance of the leukemogenic effect with time after exposure seems to differ by city. In Nagasaki, it seems very important to confirm whether or not the leukemogenic effect truly disappeared. The occurrence of leukemia in a so-called open sample of A-bomb survivors in Nagasaki was examined from 1970–78 and 2 or 3 leukemia cases per year were identified among those with exposure of 1 rad or more. Further, several cases of preleukemia were detected in the proximally exposed survivors since 1970 (*4*). In view of these facts, it may be inappropriate to say that the leukemogenic effect of A-bomb radiation has disappeared in Nagasaki, although it appears to have disappeared among the RERF sample in Nagasaki. One of the reasons for this apparent disappearance may be that the size of the RERF sample in Nagasaki is too small (15,000 survivors and 11,000 controls).

Kawakami *et al.* (*13*) reported 19 cases of leukemia that occurred during 1978–81 among A-bomb survivors who were exposed within 2,000 m from ground zero in Hiroshima and indicated that there still is a risk of A-bomb induced leukemia.

Figure 4 gives the age ATB specific annual incidence rate for all types of leukemia during 1950–78 by dose and city. The excess risk in individuals who received 100 rad or more kerma total dose did not differ significantly among four age ATB categories.

Figure 5 shows the age ATB specific annual incidence rate for all types of leukemia among individuals who received 100 rad or more kerma total dose by city and period. When the age ATB specific annual incidence rates are examined for dose and years after exposure, it is noted that the larger the excess risk among those of younger ages ATB who received 100 rad or more kerma total dose, the greater the effect of radiation in the early period and the more rapid the decline in risk up to 1960. The effect among those persons who were aged 30 years or more ATB is of lesser magnitude, but it is more

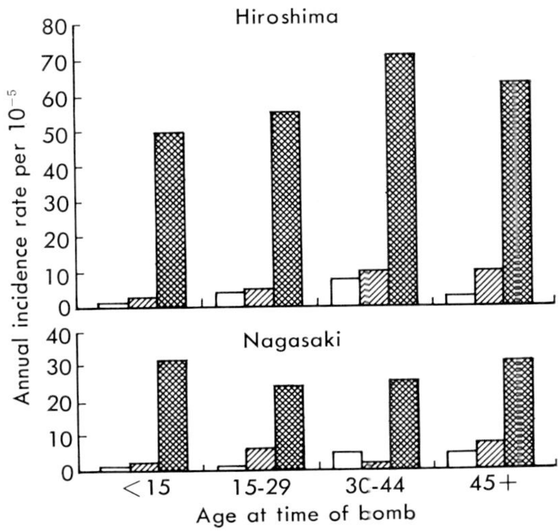

FIG. 4. Age ATB specific annual incidence rate for all types of leukemia in the RERF sample by dose, and city, 1950–78. □, control; ▨, 1–99 rad; ▩, 100+ rad.

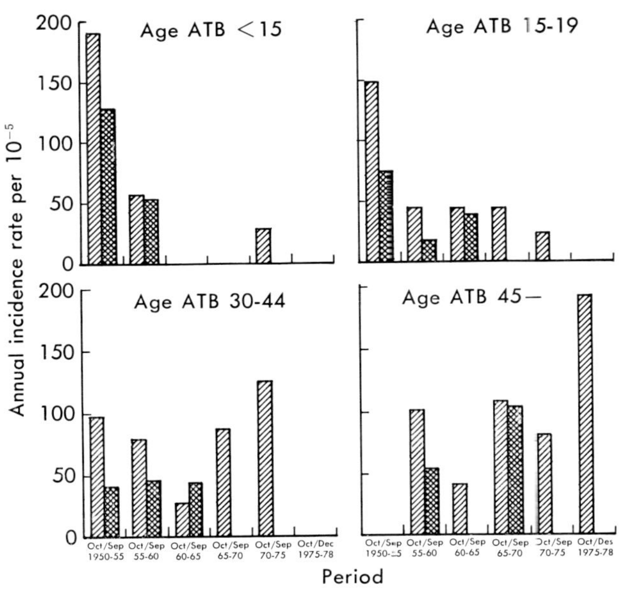

FIG. 5. Age ATB specific annual incidence rate for all types of leukemia among survivors who received 100 rad or more by time period and city, 1950–78. ▨, Hiroshima; ▩, Nagasaki.

prolonged. The effect among individuals who were aged 45 years or more ATB did not appear until 1955 (10 years after exposure) and the risk has been highest in the most recent 3 years in Hiroshima. The risk has been greater in Hiroshima than in Nagasaki for most age ATB groups and for most periods. After 1970, an excess risk in survivors in the RERF sample who received 100 rad or more kerma total dose is apparent in Hiroshima survivors whose age ATB was 30 or more. Again, the leukemogenic effect of

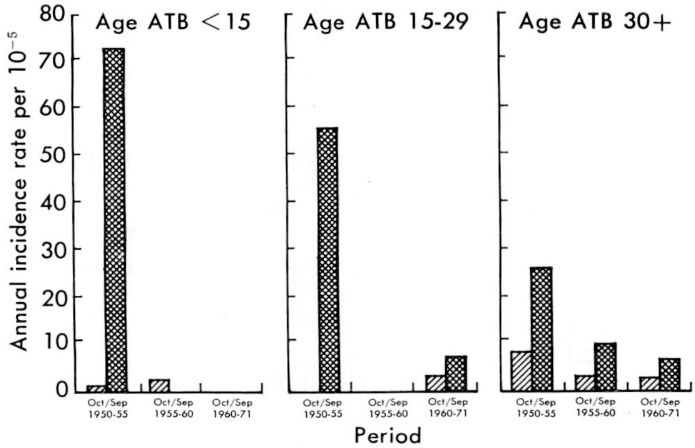

FIG. 7. Age ATB specific annual incidence rate (per 100,000 of CML among A-bomb survivors, by dose and time period, 1950–71. ▨, 1–99 rad; ▩, 100+ rad.

Typical CML with Ph[1] chromosome has not been observed in animal leukemia, so information about CML obtained from A-bomb survivors is important. Ph[1] chromosome was demonstrated in all CML patients among A-bomb survivors examined and there has been no clear difference between the features of CML among A-bomb survivors and nonexposed persons.

CML in A-bomb survivors could be found in the early phase without splenomegaly. After detailed observations of CML in A-bomb survivors, Kamada *et al.* (*11*) pointed out the progressive manifestations of CML as appearance of Ph[1] chromosome → increased basophils → elevated leukocytes → decrease of neutrophil alkaline phosphatase (NAP) → elevated serum VB_{12} → splenomegaly.

The Nishiyama district in Nagasaki is known as an area of A-bomb radioactive fallout and residents of Nishiyama were possibly exposed to low dose radiation externally as well as internally by means of the continuous intake of agricultural products during a long period. The estimated dose of only the external exposure in this area was reported to be 30 to 130 rad by Okajima. Leukocytosis of unknown cause was recognized about 2 years after the A-bomb (*5*). Later, two cases of CML occurred among residents of this area. Long-term exposure to low dose radiation is likely to induce CML.

Leukemia Among Individuals Exposed in Utero, and Children of A-Bomb Survivors

The incidence of leukemia has been analyzed in relation to the fetal dose of individuals exposed in utero, and the parental gonadal dose of individuals born to A-bomb survivors and controls in two RERF fixed samples (in utero mortality and clinical follow-up). Among 3,636 in utero exposed children and controls, 3 leukemia cases were identified through 1979 (*8*).

Table II shows the crude annual incidence rate for leukemia among the in utero exposed children and controls in Hiroshima and Nagasaki during 1945–79. There were 3 leukemia cases in this sample during the 34-year follow-up period. No excess risk for exposed children appears to exist. Only one person among those individuals who received 1 rad or more developed acute lymphocytic leukemia.

TABLE II. Crude Annual Incidence Rate for Leukemia among in Utero Exposed Children and Controls, Hiroshima and Nagasaki, 1945–79

Item		Fetus total dose in rad				Total
		NIC	0	1–49	50+	
Subjects		2,306	625	620	85	3,636
Person-years		72,444	19,403	19,078	2,255	113,180
Leukemia cases		1	1	1	0	3
Rate (10^{-5})		1.38	5.15	5.24	0.00	2.65
90% confidence limit	Upper	6.55	24.46	24.87	—	6.85
	Lower	0.07	0.27	0.27	—	0.72

Leukemia Cases

No.	MF No.	Sex	Fetus dose: Gamma	Fetus dose: Neutrons	Type of leukemia	Onset	Age at onset	Date of birth
1	848523	M	2 rad	0	Acute lymphocytic	March 1976	29	1 April 1946
2	246505	F	0	0	Acute myelogenous	July 1963	18	8 August 1945
3	442671	M	NIC		Acute, type undetermined	December 1954	9	7 December 1945

TABLE III. Crude Annual Incidence Rate for Leukemia in the F_1 Mortality Sample by Parental Gonadal Dose, Hiroshima and Nagasaki, 1946–79

Maternal dose in rad	Item		Paternal dose in rad			Total
			50+	1–49	Control[a]	
50+	Subjects		177	129	2,035	2,341
	Person-years		4,673	3,394	52,942	61,009
	Case		0	1	1	2
	Rate (10^{-5})		0.0	29.5	1.9	3.3
	90% confidence limits	Upper	—	139.8	9.0	10.3
		Lower	—	1.5	0.1	0.6
1–49	Subjects		401	1,703	7,291	9,395
	Person-years		10,678	46,983	193,926	251,587
	Case		0	0	4	4
	Rate (10^{-5})		0.0	0.0	2.1	1.6
	90% confidence limits	Upper	—	—	4.7	3.6
		Lower	—	—	0.7	0.5
Control*	Subjects		1,713	3,264	33,976	38,953
	Person-years		44,361	85,379	897,043	1,026,783
	Case		2	2	26	30
	Rate (10^{-5})		4.5	2.3	2.9	2.9
	90% confidence limits	Upper	14.2	7.4	4.0	4.0
		Lower	0.8	0.4	2.0	2.1
Total	Subjects		2,291	5,096	43,302	50,689
	Person-years		59,712	135,756	1,143,911	1,339,379
	Case		2	3	31	36
	Rate (10^{-5})		3.3	2.2	2.7	2.7
	90% confidence limits	Upper	10.6	5.7	3.7	3.6
		Lower	0.6	0.6	2.0	2.0

[a] 0 rad+not in city ATB.

Table III gives the crude annual incidence rate for leukemia among children born to exposed parents and controls in the F_1 mortality samples, Hiroshima and Nagasaki, by parental gonadal dose. In this sample 36 leukemia cases have been identified during 1946–79. There is no significant excess risk among these children where either or both parents were exposed.

Based on retrospective studies of children exposed in utero or the preconception exposure of their parents to diagnostic X-rays, a significant increased risk of leukemia in the in utero exposed and children conceived subsequent to exposure has been reported by Stewart *et al.* (*19*), McMahon (*14*), and Graham *et al.* (*3*). However, studies of A-bomb survivors show no significant excess risk of leukemia among in utero exposed children nor among children born to exposed parents.

Radiation Induced Leukemia and Chromosome Abnormality

The study of chromosomes seems to be one useful method to clarify the mechanism of radiation effects on leukemogenesis as leukemia is a disease of monoclonal proliferation of white blood cells. Even now some healthy A-bomb survivors have chromosome abnormalities in peripheral blood lymphocytes in proportion to their estimated radiation dose. Kamada (*10*) and Tomonaga (*21*) reported a significant increase of chromosome abnormalities in bone marrow cells of A-bomb survivors, and specific chromosome abnormalities have been identified in several types of leukemia. It may be possible to clarify the mechanism of radiation induced leukemia by studying the relationship of chromosome abnormalities among healthy A-bomb survivors and survivors with leu-

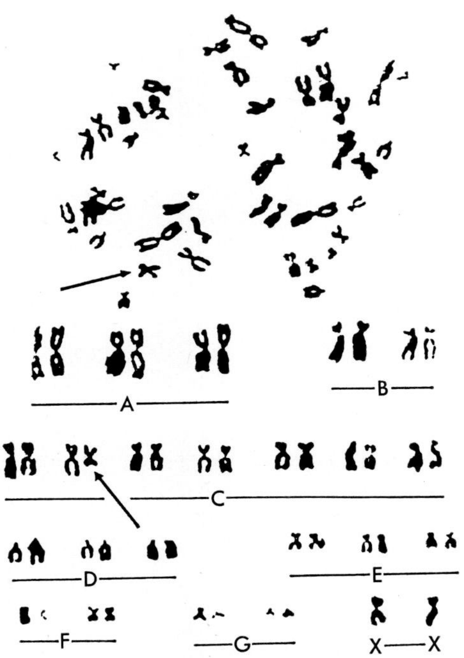

FIG. 8. Karyotype detected from colony-forming unit in culture (CFU-C) colony of proximally exposed A-bomb survivor having chromosome abnormality with 46xy, cq- (probable 7q-)

kemia. Tanaka *et al.* (*20*) reported that the chromosome break points of the T-lymphocytes of healthy A-bomb survivors are nonrandom, and relatively frequent abnormalities were observed in specific break points. The same chromosome abnormality (7q-) was found in one proximally exposed healthy survivor and a preleukemia case (probable chronic myelomonocytic leukemia) in another proximally exposed survivor (Fig. 8). Recently, Amenomori *et al.* (*1*) established a method of chromosome analysis using colony forming cells induced from hematopoietic stem cells. This method is considered useful to identify whether or not the same chromosome abnormalities seen in peripheral lymphocytes of A-bomb survivors also exist in their hematopoietic stem cells. In addition, it will be possible by this method to elucidate whether or not specific chromosome abnormalities in leukemia patients are also present in their hematopoietic stem cells.

Multiple Myeloma (*MM*)

MM is a malignancy of B-cell (plasma cell) lineage and is a relatively rare disease. Malignant cells in this disease proliferate mainly in the bone marrow. The incidence of MM among A-bomb survivors previously had not been found to be significantly elevated. On the basis of Atomic Bomb Casualty Commission (ABCC) autopsy material for 1948–62 Anderson and Ishida (*2*) reported that the incidence of MM among A-bomb survivors in Hiroshima was slightly increased in the group exposed within 1,400 m from ground zero, as compared to the incidence in those individuals exposed beyond that distance; however, there was only one MM case in the group exposed within 1,400 m. Yamamoto and Wakabayashi (*23*) reported an absence of evidence of radiation induced bone tumors, including MM, in A-bomb survivors in Hiroshima and Nagasaki during 1950–65. Nishiyama *et al.* (*18*) also studied malignant lymphoma and MM in the same fixed sample of A-bomb survivors, but they could not demonstrate a significant excess risk of MM

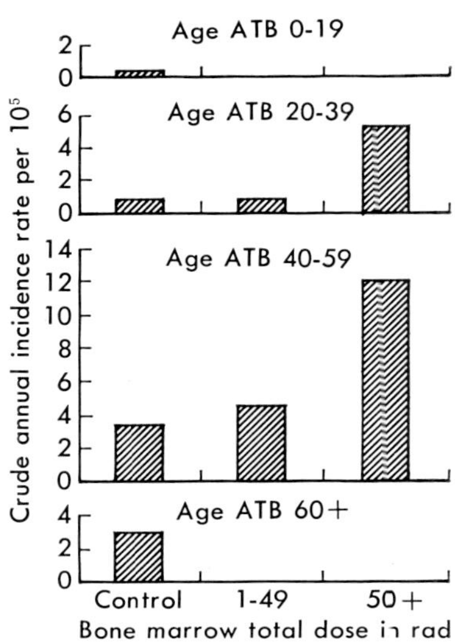

FIG. 9. Crude annual incidence rate of multiple myeloma for A-bomb survivors and controls in the RERF sample, by age ATB and total marrow dose, Hiroshima and Nagasaki, 1950–76.

in the heavily exposed. Thus, for 20 years after the A-bombs, no persuasive evidence of an excess of MM among the survivors was found.

In 1982, more than 30 years after the A-bombs, an analysis of MM incidence was conducted among A-bomb survivors and controls for the 26-year period from October 1950 to December 1976 and 29 cases of MM were identified (*6*). These 29 cases were divided into 3 bone marrow total dose classes (50+ rad, 1–49 rad, and controls) and 4 age ATB groups (0–19, 20–39, 40–59, and 60+). As shown in Fig. 9, the relative risk in those aged 20 to 59 years ATB tends to increase with dose for both sexes in both cities. When the data were divided into the 3 dose groups and 4 age ATB groups, the number of cases in each of the 12 categories was small. However, a dose effect was not evident among those individuals whose age ATB was less than 20 years or 60 or more years, although the risk tends to increase in the control group with age.

Clearly, MM occurs frequently after 50 years of age, and thus the failure to see an effect in the under 20 years group may merely reflect the fact that these individuals have not yet reached the age at which MM is more prone to develop. The apparent absence of a radiation effect among the older individuals is thought to be due to other reasons.

The size of the oldest group was small especially in the heavily exposed, and most of these individuals may have died before MM would have occurred as a radiation effect. A dose effect for MM was evident only among those individuals 20–59 years of age ATB. Observation of the under 20 age ATB group when they have reached the age of risk is suggested.

A simple graphical method called "hazard plotting" was used to compare the cumulative risk of MM in 3 dose groups in relation to years after exposure. Figure 10 shows the cumulative hazard rates for individuals aged 20–59 ATB in 3 marrow dose groups from 1950 to 1976. An increased risk in the high-dose group (50+ rad) does not

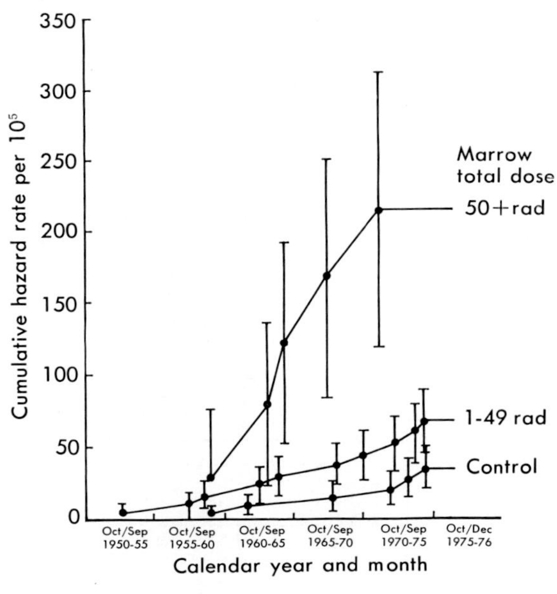

FIG. 10. Cumulative hazard rate for multiple myeloma among A-bomb survivors and controls aged 20–59 years ATB in the RERF sample, Hiroshima and Nagasaki, 1950–76.

become apparent until 20 years after exposure when the risk shows a gradual increase.

As myelomatous cells are of B-lymphocyte lineage, MM, like malignant lymphoma, seems to be a malignancy of mature lymphocytes. The carcinogenic effect for blood cells seems to differ in their differentiated level. Furthermore, some age-dependent factor may be necessary for the occurrence of MM.

The risk of MM for the under age 20 ATB group may develop in the future, and a significant increase in malignant monoclonal M-protein disease (MM and macroglobulinemia) 35 years after exposure has been confirmed again using the RERF Life Span Study (LSS) sample during October 1979–September 1981 (*16*).

Malignant Lymphoma

Anderson and Ishida (*2*) reported excess risk of malignant lymphoma including Hodgkin's disease, lymphosarcoma, reticulum cell sarcoma, and MM among Hiroshima A-bomb survivors using autopsy and surgical materials during 1949–62. Nishiyama *et al.* (*18*) also reported the same findings among Hiroshima survivors using the materials during 1945–65. The incidence of malignant lymphoma except MM was reviewed using the RERF sample during 1950–77. Table IV gives the prevalence rate of malignant lym-

TABLE IV. Prevalence Rate for Malignant Lymphoma in the RERF Sample by Dose and Type of Lymphoma, Hiroshima and Nagasaki, 1950–77

Item	Dose category (rad)					
	Control (A)	1–99 (B)	100–199 (C)	200+ (D)	Unknown	Total
Number of subjects	41,028	39,204	3,111	2,930	2,409	88,682
Average total dose (rad)	0	17.3	141.2	349.6	—	
			Number of cases			
Hodgkin's disease	10	10	2	0	0	22
Non-Hodgkin's lymphoma	45	41	3	9	1	99
Malignant lymphoma (total)	55	51	5	9	1	121
		Crude prevalence rate per 1,000 population				
Hodgkin's disease	0.24	0.26	0.64	0.00	0.00	0.25
Non-Hodgkin's lymphoma	1.10	1.05	0.96	3.07	0.42	1.12
Malignant lymphoma	1.34	1.31	1.60	3.07	0.42	1.37
Standardized relative risk	1.0	1.0	1.3	2.6		

A=(C+D) $\chi^2(1)=3.361$ $p<0.10$ suggestive.
A=(D) $\chi^2(1)=5.594$ $p<0.05$ significant.

TABLE V. Relationship between Age ATB and Year of Onset for Malignant Lymphoma Cases in the LSS Sample Who Received 200 rad or More Radiation Dose

Year of onset	Age ATB				
	0–19	20–39	40–59	60+	Total
–1950	1	0	0	0	1
1951–1960	0	1	0	1	2
1961–1970	1	2	1	0	4
1971–1977	0	2	0	0	2
Total	2	5	1	1	9

phoma in the sample by dose and type of lymphoma for Hiroshima and Nagasaki.

The crude prevalence rate of non-Hodgkin's lymphoma among survivors exposed to 200 rad or more showed a significant increase. However, there was no increase of Hodgkin's disease among A-bomb survivors. There were more malignant lymphoma cases who received 200 rad or more detected since 1960 as shown in Table V. It appears that non-Hodgkin's lymphoma increased after 1960 as well as MM.

Recently, malignant lymphoma has been divided into T- or B-cell types by surface marker study of tumor cells. It would be interesting to learn which type of malignant lymphoma was induced by A-bomb radiation. In Kyushu, the predominant occurrence of T-cell type non-Hodgkin's lymphoma was reported (7). Surface marker data are not available for study of these cases among A-bomb survivors.

REFERENCES

1. Amenomori, T., Tomonaga, M., Tomonaga, Y., Yao, E., Jinnai, I., Yoshida, Y., Kuriyama, K., Matsuo, T., Sadamori, N., and Ichimaru, M. A simple method for chromosomal preparation from individual hematopoietic colonies. *Acta Haematol. Jpn.*, **46**, 665–670 (1983) (in Japanese).
2. Anderson, R. E. and Ishida, K. Malignant lymphoma in the survivors of the atomic bomb in Hiroshima. *Ann. Intern. Med.*, **61**, 853–862 (1964).
3. Graham, S., Levin, M. L., Lilienfeld, A. M., Schuman, L. M., Gibson, R., Dowd, J. E., and Hempleman, L. Preconception, intrauterine, and postnatal irradiation as related to leukemia. *Natl. Cancer Inst. Monogr.*, **19**, 347–371 (1966).
4. Ichimaru, M. The diseases of hematopoietic organs among A-bomb survivors, Nagasaki. *Clinika*, **8**, 981–989 (1981) (in Japanese).
5. Ichimaru, M. Late effects of atomic bomb radiation in the Nishiyama district. *Hiroshima Igaku*, **29**, 294–297 (1976) (in Japanese).
6. Ichimaru, M., Ishimaru, T., Mikami, M., and Matsunaga, M. Multiple myeloma among atomic bomb survivors in Hiroshima and Nagasaki, 1950–76: Relationship to radiation dose absorbed by marrow. *J. Natl. Cancer Inst.*, **69**, 323–328 (1982).
7. Ichimaru, M., Kinoshita, K., Kamihira, S., Ikeda, S., Yamada, Y., and Amagasaki, T. T-cell malignant lymphoma in Nagasaki district and its problems. *Jpn. J. Clin. Oncol.*, **9** (Suppl.), 337–346 (1979).
8. Ishimaru, T., Ichimaru, M., and Mikami, M. Leukemia incidence among individuals exposed in utero, children of atomic bomb survivors and their controls: Hiroshima and Nagasaki, 1945–1979. RERF Tech. Rep. 11-81 (1981).
9. Ishimaru, T., Otake, M., and Ichimaru, M. Dose relationship of neutron and gamma rays to leukemia incidence among atomic bomb survivors in Hiroshima and Nagasaki by type of leukemia, 1950–1971, *Radiat. Res.*, **77**, 377–394 (1979).
10. Kamada, N. The atomic bomb and cancer—from the standpoint of chromosome aberrations. *Nagasaki Med. J.*, **47**, 356–366 (1972) (in Japanese).
11. Kamada, N., Oguma, N., Tanaka, R., Kuramoto, A., Ohkita, T., Takahashi, H., Ito, C., and Kimura, H. Development of chronic myelocytic leukemia in atomic bomb survivors. *Hiroshima Igaku*, **33**, 506–511 (1978) (in Japanese).
12. Kato, H. and Schull, W. J. Studies of the mortality of A-bomb survivors. 7, Mortality, 1950–78, Part 1. Cancer mortality. *Radiat. Res.*, **90**, 395–432 (1982).
13. Kawakami, M., Hayakawa, N., Tanaka, K., Ohkita, T., and Kurihara, N. Recent trends of A-bomb leukemia in Hiroshima, 1972–1981, and two cases of early CGL diagnosed among proximally exposed survivors. *Hiroshima Igaku*, **3**, 477–480 (1984) (in Japanese).

14. MacMahon, B. Prenatal X-ray exposure and childhood cancer. *J. Natl. Cancer Inst.*, **28**, 1178–1191 (1962).
15. Marshall, E. New A-bomb studies alter radiation estimates. *Science*, **212**, 900–903 (1981).
16. Mikami, M., Ishimaru, T., Kuramoto, A., Abe. T., Yamada, Y., Amagasaki, T., and Ichimaru, M. M-proteinemia in A-bomb survivors and controls, Hiroshima and Nagasaki, Oct. 1979– Sept. 1981. RERF Tech. Rep., in preparation.
17. Milton, R. C. and Shohoji, T. Tentative 1965 radiation dose estimation for atomic bomb survivors, Hiroshima and Nagasaki. ABCC Tech. Rep. 1-68 (1968).
18. Nishiyama, H., Anderson, R. E., Ishimaru, T., Ishida, K., Ii, Y., and Okabe, N. The incidence of malignant lymphoma and multiple myeloma in Hiroshima and Nagasaki atomic bomb survivors, 1945–65. *Cancer*, **32**, 1301–1309 (1973).
19. Stewart, A., Webb, J., and Hewitt, D. A survey of childhood malignancies. *Br. Med. J.*, **1**, 1495–1508 (1958).
20. Tanaka, K., Kamada, N., Ohkita, T., and Kuramoto, A. Chromosome break points in T-lymphocytes from atomic bomb survivors: Comparison with specific chromosome aberrations found in leukemia. *Hiroshima Iagaku*, **35**, 1214–1221 (1982) (in Japanese).
21. Tomonaga, Y. Chromosome abnormalities in atomic bomb survivors. *Nagasaki Med. J.*, **51**, 282–286 (1976) (in Japanese).
22. Watanabe, S. Cancer and leukemia developing among atom-bomb survivors, Geshwulste, Tumors I (Handbuch der allgemeinen Pathologie, Vol. 5), ed. by E. Grundmann, pp. 461–577 (1974). Springer-Verlag, Berlin.
23. Yamamoto, T., and Wakabayashi, T. Bone tumors among the atomic bomb survivors of Hiroshima and Nagasaki. *Acta Pathol. Jpn.*, **19**, 201–212 (1969).

gland cancer among A-bomb survivors. In a subsequent study on the AHS population the incidence of salivary gland tumors was 9.3-fold higher in the group exposed to 300+ rad than in the control group and when confined only to malignant tumors the incidence was 21.8-fold higher.

Thyroid

Reports on thyroid cancer in Hiroshima and Nagasaki atomic bomb (A-bomb) survivors can be traced back to the 1950s. Kaneko and Numata (*10*) reported in 1957 a case of thyroid cancer which developed with leukemia in a 12-year old girl exposed to A-bomb radiation at a distance of 800 m from ground zero in Hiroshima, and in 1959 Fujimoto *et al.* (*5*, *6*) reported three cases of thyroid cancer in A-bomb survivors.

In 1963 Hollingsworth *et al.* (*8*) made a systematic analysis of thyroid gland diseases in a population of survivors and suggested the presence of a tendency for the incidence of thyroid cancer to be high among A-bomb survivors. They studied 12 thyroid cancer cases found in the AHS population during 1958–59 and suggested that the incidence of thyroid cancer was high among proximally exposed (within 1,500 m from ground zero) survivors, especially among females. The study was continued on the same population, and Socolow *et al.* (*14*), making an analysis in 1963 on 21 cases of thyroid cancer identified during the 3-year period 1958–61, confirmed that the incidence of thyroid cancer was high among A-bomb survivors proximally exposed. Wood *et al.* (*19*) reported similar results in 1968, in which they studied the relationship between radiation dose and thyroid cancer incidence among survivors exposed within 2,000 m from ground zero and demonstrated a tendency for the incidence to be elevated with increased dose. Parker *et al.* (*11*) summarized a 1958–71 study on the same population. According to their summarization, the number of cases of thyroid cancer identified during this period was 74, and the incidence was high in the 50+ rad group, especially in females exposed at under 20 years of age. Of the 74 cases 34 were found only at postmortem examination. Minute cancer was found at a high frequency at autopsy, and it is known that most such cancer does not develop into malignancies which would become clinically apparent. If the analysis is made including minute cancer found at autopsy, the incidence will become elevated but no longer be applicable to clinical experience.

Members of the LSS sample, a larger ABCC-RERF study population, are included in the ABCC-RERF autopsy program. During 1957–68 autopsies were conducted on 3,067 cases, and Sampson *et al.* (*12*, *13*) made detailed examinations on the thyroid glands of these cases and found thyroid cancer in 536 cases. Of these cases 518 (96.6%) were occult cancer less than 1.5 cm in size. Analysis of these 536 cases showed increased thyroid cancer prevalence in A-bomb survivors exposed to 50+ rad.

Reports have been made on thyroid cancer among survivors studied in other study populations, but these are not fixed populations. Ezaki and Shigematsu (*3*) studied the incidence of thyroid cancer in patients seen in the outpatient clinic of the Department of Surgery, Hiroshima University School of Medicine, and found it to be 2.25% (38/1,509) and significantly higher in those exposed to A-bomb radiation as compared to 0.44% (58/13,211) for the nonexposed. The incidence of thyroid cancer in the exposed was higher in females, with 32 of 38 cases being females as against 6 males. Six of the 38 cases (15.8%) were A-bomb survivors proximally exposed within 1,000 m from ground zero indicating that thyroid cancer incidence is high among them. Further, 7 of the 38 cases were so-called early entrants who entered the city within two weeks after the bombing.

Ezaki and Shigematsu (*3*) studied thyroid cancer incidence among those insured under the national health insurance program in Hiroshima City during 1960–61 in order to observe the tendency in Hiroshima City as a whole, and the incidence in A-bomb survivors (26.80 per 100,000 population) was found to be almost 5-fold that in the nonexposed (5.25 per 100,000 population). Harano *et al.* (*7*) studied 394 cases of thyroid gland diseases operated on and histopathologically diagnosed in Nagasaki City by 1965 and found 116 cases of thyroid cancer. Since 42 of these cases were exposed to the A-bomb and 74 were controls (43.6% exposed and 24.8% nonexposed) they reported that thyroid cancer incidence was higher in the exposed.

Among the study samples established to date, ABCC-RERF studies have been made mainly on the sample composed of 20,000 AHS subjects, but this population is small for conducting epidemiological studies. On the other hand, the populations of other studies have the disadvantage of not being fixed populations and having no radiation dose estimation made for them. Overcoming these disadvantages, Ezaki (*4*) studied and analyzed data on thyroid cancer diagnosed or detected at autopsy during the 22 years from 1958 to 1979, in a sample of 75,493 study subjects exposed in Hiroshima belonging to the LSS Extended sample, excluding those whose exposure dose was unknown and those who had thyroid cancer from before 1958.

In past studies, clinically detected thyroid cancer and occult (minute) thyroid cancer were reported together, but in this study they are discussed separately because they differ greatly in character. There were 332 subjects in the population suspected of having thyroid cancer, and they were examined individually for identification. As a result, 125 cases of clinical thyroid cancer and 159 cases of occult thyroid cancer were detected.

1. *Clinical thyroid cancer*

The histopathological distribution of the 103 cases for which tissue specimens were obtained is shown in Table I. Most were papillary cancer, with no difference by exposure status. The 125 cases were composed of 15 males and 110 females, distributed by age at the time of the bomb (ATB) and exposure dose, as shown in Table II and Fig. 1;

TABLE I. Distribution of Histological Type of Clinical Thyroid Cancer Cases Whose Tissue Specimens were Obtained, Hiroshima, 1958–79

Morphologic type of carcinoma	Tissue total dose in rad			
	Control	1–49	50+	Total
Papillary	43 (100.0)	38 (90.5)	16 (88.9)	97 (94.2)
Sclerosing	0	0	0	0
Follicular	0	2 (4.8)	1 (5.6)	3 (2.9)
Epidermoid	0	1 (2.4)	0	1 (1.0)
Anaplastic	0	1 (2.4)	1 (5.6)	2 (2.0)
Medullary	0	0	0	0
Total	43 (100.0)	42 (100.1)	18 (100.1)	103 (100.1)

Percentage in parentheses.

TABLE II. Crude Annual Incidence Rates for Clinical Thyroid Cancer per 100,000 Population by Sex and Tissue Total Dose, Hiroshima 1958–79

Item	Thyroid tissue total dose in rad				
	Control	1–49	50–99	100+	Total
			Male		
Subjects	18,842	9,977	797	798	30,414
Average dose	0.0	9.1	71.2	205.6	—
Person-years	351,551	184,857	14,259	14,245	564,912
Cases	9	3	2	1	15
Rate (10^{-5})	2.6	1.6	14.0	7.0	2.7
			Female		
Subjects	28,200	14,578	1,182	1,119	45,079
Average dose	0.0	10.1	69.2	197.2	—
Person-years	554,902	284,995	23,143	21,840	884,880
Cases	46	48	7	9	110
Rate (10^{-5})	8.2	16.8	30.2	41.2	12.4

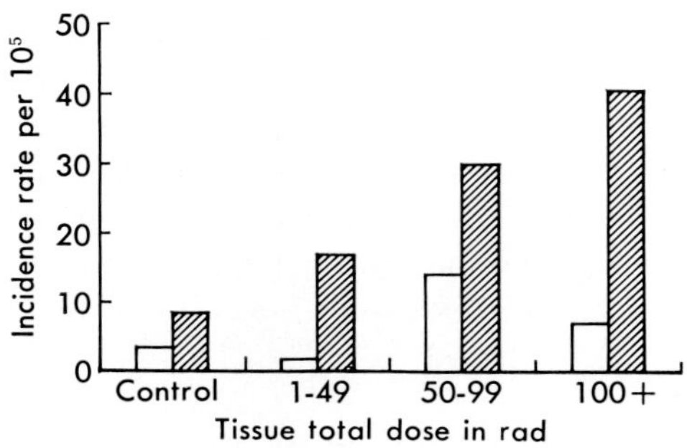

FIG. 1. Crude annual incidence rates for clinical cancer per 100,000 population by sex and tissue total dose. □, male; ▨, female.

and the crude annual incidence per 100,000 population was 2.7 for males and 12.4 for females. The risk of thyroid cancer in females and in both sexes combined increased with increase of dose. The increase in the high dose group is not remarkable in males, but this may be due to their small number. In males too the trend is for risk to increase with radiation dose, but this trend is not statistically significant, given the small number of cases. In females the crude annual incidence rate shows an increase of risk with increase of dose in every age group, and this tendency was particularly evident in those exposed at a young age (Table III).

When observed and expected numbers were calculated and ratios of observed to expected (O/E) sought, either by sex or sexes combined, the incidence of thyroid cancer was found to increase with increased dose. When tests of linear response were made by Mantel's statistical method to determine the presence or absence of a dose effect, a statistically significant relation was observed in females and in males and females combined. No relation could be demonstrated in males because there were few male thyroid cancer cases (Table IV). The O/E ratio showed a tendency to increase with exposure dose in every age ATB group, and this was especially remarkable in those under 20 years of age. Tests of linear response, which shows dose effect, showed it to be statistically

TABLE III. Age ATB Specific Annual Incidence Rates for Clinical Thyroid Cancer by Tissue Total Dose and Sex, Hiroshima 1958–79

Age ATB	Item	Tissue total dose in rad				Total	Tissue total dose in rad				Total
		Control	1–49	50–99	100+		Control	1–49	50–99	100+	
				Male					Female		
0–9	PY[a]	100,210	51,009	3,067	2,647	156,933	103,048	52,737	3,445	2,994	162,224
	Cases	1	0	0	1	2	4	5	1	1	11
	Rate (10^{-5})	1.00	0.00	0.00	37.78	1.27	3.88	9.48	29.03	33.40	6.78
10–19	PY	90,006	48,884	3,494	4,185	146,569	118,766	57,500	5,626	5,903	187,795
	Cases	3	0	1	0	4	8	9	2	4	23
	Rate (10^{-5})	3.33	0.00	28.62	0.00	2.73	6.74	15.65	35.55	67.76	12.25
20–29	PY	31,554	16,403	1,322	1,851	50,930	105,998	55,155	4,984	4,920	171,057
	Cases	3	0	0	0	3	16	6	1	1	24
	Rate (10^{-5})	9.51	0.00	0.00	0.00	5.89	15.10	10.88	20.06	20.33	14.03
30–39	PY	48,864	24,389	2,399	2,011	77,663	104,156	55,255	3,903	3,771	167,085
	Cases	1	1	0	0	2	6	12	1	2	21
	Rate (10^{-5})	2.05	4.10	0.00	0.00	2.58	5.76	21.72	25.62	53.04	12.57
40–49	PY	53,129	28,279	2,664	2,257	86,329	80,170	42,132	3,572	3,193	129,065
	Cases	1	1	0	0	2	9	11	1	1	22
	Rate (10^{-5})	1.88	3.54	0.00	0.00	2.32	11.23	26.11	28.00	31.34	17.05
50+	PY	27,989	15,893	1,313	1,293	46,488	42,763	22,215	1,612	1,063	67,854
	Cases	0	1	1	0	2	3	5	1	0	9
	Rate (10^{-5})	0.00	6.29	76.16	0.00	4.30	7.02	22.51	62.04	0.00	13.30
Total	PY	351,552	184,857	14,259	14,244	554,912	554,901	234,995	23,142	21,842	884,880
	Cases	9	3	2	1	15	45	48	7	9	110
	Rate (10^{-5})	2.55	1.62	14.03	7.02	2.66	8.29	16.84	30.25	41.21	12.43
				Both sexes							
Total	PY	906,453	469,852	37,401	35,086	1,449,792					
	Cases	55	51	9	10	125					
	Rate (10^{-5})	6.07	10.85	24.06	27.71	8.62					
Standardized incidence rate (10^{-5})		5.62	10.02	25.42	20.30	7.92					

Standard incidence rate adjusted for sex and age ATB.

[a] Person-years.

TABLE IV. Comparison of Observed and Expected Number of Clinical Thyroid Cancer Cases by Tissue Total Dose and Sex, Hiroshima 1958–79

Item	Tissue total dose in rad					Test for linearity χ^2 [1] p
	Control	1–49	50–99	100+	Total	
Average dose in rad	0	9.7	70.0	200.7	—	
			Total			
Subjects	47,042	24,555	1,979	1,917	75,493	
Observed	55	51	9	10	125	26.46
Expected	78.05	40.53	3.28	3.14	125.00	$p<0.001$***
O/E	0.70	1.26	2.74	3.18	1.00	
			Male			
Subjects	18,843	9,977	797	798	30,414	
Observed	9	3	2	1	15	2.70
Expected	9.30	4.90	0.40	0.40	15.00	$p<0.10$ NS
O/E	0.97	0.61	5.00	2.50	1.00	
			Female			
Subjects	28,200	14,578	1,182	1,119	45,079	
Observed	46	48	7	8	110	23.81
Expected	68.75	35.63	2.88	2.74	110.00	$p<0.001$***
O/E	0.67	1.35	2.43	3.28	1.00	

Expected number adjusted for age ATB.
NS (Not significant), $0.10<p$; $0.05<p\leqslant0.10$; * $0.01<p\leqslant0.05$; ** $0.001<p\leqslant0.01$; *** $p\leqslant0.001$.

TABLE V. Comparison of Observed and Expected Number of Clinical Thyroid Cancer Cases by Tissue Total Dose and Age ATB, Hiroshima 1958–79

Item	Tissue total dose in rad					Test for linearity χ^2 [1] p
	Control	1–49	50–99	100+	Total	
Average dose in rad	0	9.7	70.0	200.7	—	
			Age ATB: under 20			
Subjects	19,060	9,733	731	745	30,274	
Observed	16	14	4	6	40	34.64
Expected	25.27	12.69	1.02	1.02	40.00	$p<0.001$***
O/E	0.63	1.10	3.92	5.88	1.00	
			Age ATB: 20–39			
Subjects	14,084	7,355	609	627	22,575	
Observed	26	19	2	3	50	2.88
Expected	31.03	16.30	1.32	1.35	50.00	$0.10<p<0.05$
O/E	0.84	1.17	1.52	2.22	1.00	
			Age ATB: 40 and over			
Subjects	13,398	7,462	639	545	22,544	
Observed	13	18	3	1	35	1.91
Expected	21.75	11.54	0.94	0.77	35.00	$p>0.10$ NS
O/E	0.60	1.56	3.19	1.30	1.00	

Expected number adjusted for sex

significant in those under age 20 ATB, suggestive in those 20–39, and unclear in those 40 and over, with dose effect more evident the younger the age (Table V). The relative risk of thyroid cancer in the 50+ rad group as compared to the control group and the

TABLE VI. Standardized Relative Risk of Clinical Thyroid Cancer, 50+ rad *vs.* Control, Hiroshima 1958–79

Dose group	Subjects	Cases	Statistical test χ^2 [*d.f.* = 1]	Standardized relative risk	95% confidence limits
		Total (adjusted for sex and age ATB)			
50+ rad	3,896	19	31.96	4.2	6.9–2.6
Control	47,042	55	$p<0.001$***	1.0	
		Male (adjusted for age ATB)			
50+ rad	1,595	3	2.92	4.0	19.3–0.8
Control	18,842	9	Suggestive $0.05<p<0.10$	1.0	
		Female (adjusted for age ATB)			
50+ rad	2,301	16	26.89	4.3	7.3–2.5
Control	28,200	46	$p<0.001$***	1.0	
		Age ATB: 0–19 (adjusted for sex)			
50+ rad	1,476	10	32.32	7.9	16.1–3.9
Control	19,060	16	$p<0.001$***	1.0	
		Age ATB: 20–39 (adjusted for sex)			
50+ rad	1,236	5	1.83	2.2	7.1–0.7
Control	14,084	26	$p>0.10$ NS	1.0	
		Age ATB: 40+(adjusted for sex)			
50+ rad	1,184	4	4.50	4.0	14.2–1.1
Control	13,898	13	$p<0.05$*	1.0	

Mantel-Haenszel test procedure.

results of tests of the statistical significance of the differences are shown in Table VI. The relative risk with standardization for sex and age ATB was 4.2 (6.9–2.6 at 95% confidence limits). There was no difference of risk by sex, and the risk in males was not statistically significant because of the small number of male cases. The risk by age ATB was 7.9 in the under 20 group, 2.2 in the 20–39 group, and 4.0 in the 40 and over group, and statistically significant difference was observed only in the under 20 group (Table VI). The increase of risk per rad, which was calculated only for females under 20 whose data conformed to the model and for whom significant regression coefficients were obtained statistically, was approximately 3.4 per year per 1,000,000 population.

2. *Occult thyroid cancer*

Occult thyroid cancer was detected in 155 cases (3.5%) of the 4,425 cases autopsied during the same period. Compared to the control group, the relative risk in the 50+ rad group was significantly elevated at 1.9 (Table VII). Observed by sex and exposure dose, both males and females present no difference from the control group in the 1–40 rad

TABLE VII. Relative Risk of Occult Thyroid Cancer at Autopsy *vs.* Controls, Hiroshima 1958–79

Dose group	Autopsies	Cases	Standardized relative risk[a] (95% confidence limits)
50+ rad	341	21	1.9 (1.1–3.2)
Control	2,495	82	1.0

Mantel-Haenszel test: $\chi^2=5.35$, *d.f.* = 1, $p<0.05$.

[a] Adjusted for sex and age at death (<50, 50–59, 60–69, 70–79, and 80+).

TABLE VIII. Comparison of Observed and Expected Number of Occult Thyroid Cancer Cases by Tissue Total Dose and Sex, Hiroshima 1958–79

Item	Tissue total dose in rad			Total
	Control	1–49	50+	
Average dose in rad	0	9.7	134.3	
		Male		
Subjects	1,303	762	168	2,233
Observed	32	17	7	56
Expected	32.9	18.8	4.3	56.0
O/E	1.0	0.9	1.5	1.0
		Female		
Subjects	1,192	827	173	2,192
Observed	50	35	14	99
Expected	53.9	37.2	7.9	99.0
O/E	0.9	0.9	1.8	1.0

Test for significance: Male, $\chi^2=1.76$, $d.f.=1$, $p>0.10$ NS; Female, $\chi^2=5.30$, $d.f.=1$, $p<0.05$*.
Expected number adjusted for age at death.

group, but show a nearly 2-fold higher prevalence in the 50+ rad group (Table VIII). What attracted attention in this study was that there was no difference in prevalence by age at death both in the exposed and the nonexposed; in other words, occult cancer occurred under 50 years of age and increased little thereafter (Table IX).

While there are objections to simply totaling the results of Hiroshima and Nagasaki where the conditions differ, in the unpublished data of Ishimaru *et al.* (*9*) the results of a study made in Nagasaki for the same period and by the same method as the study in Hiroshima have been reviewed together with the Hiroshima results. The number of study subjects in Nagasaki is 22,951, less than one third of the number in Hiroshima, but the results of Nagasaki alone were nearly the same as the results of Hiroshima. Therefore, the results combining the two cities give nearly the same conclusion as the results of Hiroshima alone.

Salivary Gland

Reports on salivary gland tumors in Hiroshima and Nagasaki A-bomb survivors began to appear at the beginning of the 1970s. Takeichi *et al.* (*16*) reported 18 cases of salivary gland tumor observed at the Hiroshima University Research Institute for Nuclear Medicine and Biology at the Hiroshima Surgical meeting in 1971. They anticipated that the incidence of such tumors would be high and the frequency of the malignant types of those tumors high in A-bomb survivors, and prepared a report of their findings in 1976. In 1972, Belsky *et al.* (*1*) made the first screening on the AHS population and found 22 cases of salivary gland tumors including 8 malignant cases during 1957–70, and they observed the incidence of both types of tumors to be elevated with increased exposure dose.

Extending their study later, Takeichi *et al.* (*15*, *17*, *18*) made an analysis on 211 cases of salivary gland tumor of definite diagnosis provided by hospitals in Hiroshima and Kure during 1953–71. Among those living in Hiroshima at the time of diagnosis, 36 cases of salivary gland tumor occurred among the exposed and 30 among the non-

TABLE IX. Prevalence of Occult Thyroid Cancer at Autopsy by Sex, Tissue Total Dose, and Age at Death, Hiroshima 1958–79

Age at death	Tissue total dose in rad									Total		
	Control			1–49			50+					
	Average 0			Average 9.7			Average 134.3					
	Subjects	Cases	Rate	Subjects	Cases	Rate	Subjects	Cases	Rate	Subjects	Cases	Rate
Male												
<50	113	3	2.7	68	3	4.4	19	2	10.5	200	8	4.0
50–59	117	3	2.6	65	0	0.0	21	2	9.5	203	5	2.5
60–69	395	9	2.3	117	7	4.0	39	1	2.6	611	17	2.8
70–79	445	14	3.1	291	6	2.1	61	2	3.3	797	22	2.8
80+	233	3	1.3	161	1	0.6	28	0	0.0	422	4	0.9
Total	1,303	32	2.5	762	17	2.2	168	7	4.2	2,233	56	2.5
Female												
<50	72	2	2.8	54	2	3.7	23	2	8.7	149	6	4.0
50–59	119	5	4.2	79	4	5.1	19	0	0.0	217	9	4.1
60–69	251	16	6.1	173	7	4.0	39	5	12.8	473	28	5.9
70–79	404	17	4.2	286	12	3.2	61	5	8.2	751	34	4.5
80+	336	10	3.0	235	10	4.3	31	2	6.5	602	22	3.7
Total	1,192	50	4.2	827	35	4.2	173	14	8.1	2,192	99	4.5

Rate per 100 subjects.

TABLE X. Incidence of Salivary Gland Tumors by Exposure Status, Hiroshima 1953–71

Group	Total exposed	Directly exposed	Early entrants	Non-exposed
Person-years	1,729,271	1,490,146	239,125	4,333,814
All tumors				
Observed	36	31	5	30
Expected	18.82	15.61	1.83	
Test[a]	$p<0.001$	$p<0.001$	$p<0.02$	
Crude incidence[b]	2.1	2.1	2.1	0.7
Standardized incidence[c]	1.8	1.9	1.4	0.7
Malignant tumors				
Observed	19	17	2	5
Expected	6.27	5.12	0.26	
Test[a]	$p<0.001$	$p<0.001$	$p<0.001$	
Crude incidence[b]	1.1	1.1	0.8	0.1
Standardized incidence[c]	1.0	1.0	0.6	0.1
Benign tumors				
Observed	17	14	3	25
Expected	11.98	9.98	1.46	
Test[a]	$p>0.05$	$p>0.05$	$p>0.05$	
Crude incidence[b]	1.0	0.9	1.3	0.6
Standardized incidence[c]	0.9	0.9	0.8	0.5

[a] Exposed *vs.* nonexposed.
[b] Crude incidence per 100,000 per year.
[c] Rates are standardized to the age distribution of the 1960 National Census in 5-year age groups.

TABLE XI. Incidence of Salivary Gland Tumors by Exposure Distance, Hiroshima 1953–71

Group	Distance from ground zero in meters			Total	χ^2-test
	0–1,500	1,501–5,000	5,000+ (nonexposed)		
Person-years	322,768	1,167,373	4,333,814	5,823,955	
All tumors					
Observed	14	17	30	61	
Expected	3.38	12.23	45.39	61.00	$p<0.001$
Crude incidence[a]	4.3	1.5	0.7		
Standardized incidence[b]	3.8	1.3	0.7		
Malignant tumors					
Observed	7	10	5	22	
Expected	1.22	4.41	16.37	22.00	$p<0.001$
Crude incidence[a]	2.2	0.9	0.1		
Standardized incidence[b]	2.2	0.7	0.1		
Benign tumors					
Observed	7	7	25	39	
Expected	2.16	7.82	29.02	39.00	$p<0.01$
Crude incidence[a]	2.2	0.6	0.6		
Standardized incidence[b]	1.6	0.6	0.5		

[a] Crude incidence per 100,000 per year.
[b] Rates are standardized to the age distribution of the 1960 National Census in 5-year age groups.

exposed. The exposed cases included 31 cases directly exposed to A-bomb radiation within 5,000 m from ground zero and 5 so-called early entrants who entered the city within 2 weeks after the bomb and stayed in the vicinity of ground zero. The standardized

TABLE XII. Incidence of Salivary Gland Tumors by Age ATB and Exposure Distance, Hiroshima 1953–71

Exposure distance	Age in years					
	0–19		20–49		50+	
	Cases	Incidence	Cases	Incidence	Cases	Incidence
0–1,500 m	5	4.9	8	4.2	1	2.2
1,501–5,000 m	4	1.0	8	1.4	5	3.4
5,000+m (nonexposed)	19	0.6	10	0.7	1	1.3

Crude incidence per 100,000 per year.

annual incidence per 100,000 population for the exposed cases in Hiroshima was 1.9 which is 2.7-fold higher than the 0.7 for the 30 nonexposed cases, and for the early entrants it was 1.4 which is 2-fold higher than that of the nonexposed. The difference was more apparent for malignant tumors, the incidence for the directly exposed cases being 10-fold higher and that for the early entrants being 6-fold higher than that for the nonexposed cases (Table X). Classified by exposure distance into cases proximally exposed within 1,500 m from ground zero, cases distally exposed at 1,500–5,000 m, and cases nonexposed at more than 5000 m, the annual incidence per 100,000 population was 3.8 for the proximally exposed, 1.3 for the distally exposed, and 0.7 for the nonexposed, with the incidence showing a tendency to be higher the closer to ground zero. The tendency was marked in the malignant tumors (Table XI). Studying the relationship to exposure distance by age ATB, the incidence of salivary gland tumors in those 19 and under and 20–49 was found to show a tendency to increase with decrease of exposure distance, the crude incidence being a very high 4.9 per year per 100,000 population in those proximally exposed at age 19 and under ATB (Table XII). The histopathological diagnoses of all salivary gland tumors collected by Takeichi *et al.* (*15*, *17*, *18*) are shown by exposure in Table XIII.

Since 8 cases detected in the study belonged to the population reported previously by Belsky *et al.* (*1*), Belsky *et al.* (*2*) made a reanalysis of the 30 salivary gland tumor cases in the fixed population adding these 8 cases. As a result, it was found that the incidence rate for salivary gland tumors was high among those exposed to 300+ rad, and that the relative risk was compared to their controls (those not in the city (NIC) ATB and the 0 rad exposed) was as high as 9.35, and that for malignant tumors taken alone was a high 21.8 (Table XIV).

TABLE XIII. Histological Type of Salivary Gland Tumors 1950–71

Tumor	Exposed cases					Nonexposed cases				
	Parotid	Sub-maxillary	Sub-lingual	Minor	Total	Parotid	Sub-maxillary	Sub-lingual	Minor	Total
Benign tumor	26	5	0	0	31	66 (12)	21 (6)	0	6 (3)	93 (21)
	[1]				[1]	[10]	[3] [1]		[1]	[14] [(1)]
Benign mixed tumor	18	4	—	—	22	57 (10)	21 6	—	6 (3)	84 (19)
						[10]	[3] [(1)]		[1]	[14] [(1)]
Papillary cystadanomata lymphomatosa	5	1	—	—	6	6 (1)	— —	—	— —	6 (1)
Oxyphilic adenoma	—	—	—	—	—	2 —	— —	—	— —	2
Other adenoma	1		—	—	1	— (1)	— —	—	— —	(1)
	[1]				[1]					
Benign lymphoepithelial lesion	2[a]	—	—	—	2	1 —	— —	—	— —	1 —
Malignant tumor	17	9	1	4	31	19 (1)	7 —	2	3 —	31 (1)
						[3]	[1]	[1]		[5]
Malignant mixed tumor	5	4	1	1	11	5 —	2 —	1	1 —	9 —
						[1]		[1]		[2]
Mucoepidermoid tumor	5	1	—	1	7	6 (1)	2 —	1	— —	9 (1)
							[1]			[1]
Squamous cell carcinoma	1	1	—	—	2	2 —	—	—	— —	2 —
						[1]				[1]
Adenocarcinoma										
Adenoid cystic	1	3	—	1	5	2 —	1 —	—	1 —	4 —
Acinic cell	1	—	—	1	2	1 —	1 —	—	— —	2 —
Mucous cell	—	—	—	—	—	1 —	1 —	—	— —	2 —
Miscellaneous form	4	—	—	—	4	2 —	— —	—	1 —	3 —
						[1]				[1]
Total	43	14	1	4	62	85 (13)	28 (6)	2	9 (3)	124 (22)
	[1]				[1]	[13]	[4] [(1)]	[1]	[1]	[19] [(1)]

( ) Tumor cases in persons born after the A-bomb.
[ ] Tumor cases in residents outside of Hiroshima Prefecture.
[a] Bilateral case developed in one patient.

TABLE XIV. Salivary Gland Neoplasms Following Atomic Radiation

Item	Tentative 1965 dose in rad			Total
	NIC+0	1–299	300+	
Population	57,859	40,457	1,340	99,656
Person-years	700,552	487,669.5	16,171.5	1,204,393
All cases				
Observed	14	13	3	30
Expected	17.45	12.15	0.40	30.00
Relative risk	1.00	1.33	9.35	
Malignant cases				
Observed	4	3	2	9
Expected	5.23	3.64	0.12	9.00
Relative risk	1.00	1.08	21.8	

REFERENCES

1. Belsky, J. L., Tachikawa, K., Cihak, R. W., and Yamamoto, T. Salivary gland tumors in atomic bomb survivors, Hiroshima-Nagasaki, 1957–1970. *J. Am. Med. Assoc.*, **219**, 864–868 (1972).
2. Belsky, J. L., Takeichi, N., Yamamoto, T., Cihak, R. W., Hirose, F., Ezaki, H., Inoue, S., and Blot, W. J. Salivary gland neoplasms following atomic radiation: Additional cases and reanalysis of combined data in a fixed population, 1957–1970. *Cancer*, **35**, 555–559 (1975).
3. Ezaki, H. and Shigemitsu, T. Studies on thyroid cancer induced by A-bomb exposure and its clinical characteristics. *J. Hiroshima Med. Assoc.*, **20** (Suppl.), 336–347 (1967); *Proc. Hiroshima Univ. Res. Inst. Nucl. Med. Biol.*, **11**, 166–168 (1970) (in Japanese).
4. Ezaki, H. Thyroid carcinoma after exposure to atomic bomb radiation, Hiroshima 1958–79. *J. Jpn. Pract. Surg. Soc.*, **44**, 1127–1137 (1983) (in Japanese).
5. Fujimoto, Y., Yamamoto, T., Numata, J., and Mori, K. Two autopsy cases of thyroid cancer in young atomic bomb survivors. *J. Hiroshima Med. Assoc.*, **12**, 519–524 (1959) (in Japanese).
6. Fujimoto, Y., Yamamoto, T., Ishida, J., and Numata, J. Three autopsy cases of myelogenous leukemia complicated with thyroid gland tumors detected in atomic bomb survivors. *J. Hiroshima Med Assoc.*, **12**, 1077 (1959) (in Japanese).
7. Harano, A., Tezuka, H., and Shirabe, R. Thyroid gland—Study of thyroid gland diseases in atomic bomb survivors. *J. Hiroshima Med. Assoc.*, **20** (Suppl.), 336–347 (1967) (in Japanese).
8. Hollingsworth, D. R., Hamilton, H. B., Tamagaki, H., and Beebe, G. W. Thyroid disease: A study in Hiroshima, Japan. *Medicine*, **42**, 47–71 (1963).
9. Ishimaru, T., Ezaki, H., Asano, M., Fujikura, T., Nishida, T., and Izumi, M. Incidence of thyroid cancer among atomic bomb survivors and controls, Hiroshima and Nagasaki, 1958–1979: Relationship to radiation dose absorbed by thyroid gland. (unpublished data).
10. Kaneko, N. and Numata, J. An autopsy case of atomic radiation-induced leukemia complicated with thyroid gland tumor. *J. Pediatr. Pract.*, **20**, 478 (1957) (in Japanese).
11. Parker, L. N., Belsky, J. L., Yamamoto, T., Kawamoto, C., and Keehn, R. J. Thyroid carcinoma after exposure to atomic radiation: A continuing survey of a fixed population, Hiroshima and Nagasaki, 1958–1971. *Ann. Intern. Med.*, **80**, 600–604 (1974).
12. Sampson, R. J., Key, C. R., Buncher, C. R., and Iijima, S. Thyroid carcinoma in Hiro-

shima and Nagasaki, I. Prevalence of thyroid carcinoma at autopsy. *J. Am. Med. Assoc.*, **209**, 65–70 (1969).

13. Sampson, R. J., Key, C. R., Buncher, C. R., Oka, H., and Iijima, S. Papillary carcinoma of the thyroid gland, sizes of 525 tumors found at autopsy in Hiroshima and Nagasaki. *Cancer*, **25**, 1391–1393 (1970).
14. Socolow, E. L., Hashizume, A., Neriishi, S., and Niitani, R. Thyroid carcinoma in man after exposure to ionizing radiation. A summary of the findings in Hiroshima and Nagasaki. *New Engl. J. Med.*, **268**, 406–410 (1963).
15. Takeichi, N., Inoue, S., Niimoto, M., Nagata, N., and Ezaki, H. Parotid gland tumors, especially in relation to radiation exposure. *J. Jpn. Surg. Soc.*, **74**, 1170–1172 (1973) (in Japanese).
16. Takeichi, N., Hirose, F., Inoue, S., Niimoto, M., and Hattori, T. Parotid gland tumors observed at Research Institute for Nuclear Medicine and Biology, Hiroshima Univeristy. *Jpn. J. Cancer Clin.*, **22**, 307–311 (1976) (in Japanese).
17. Takeichi, N., Hirose, F., and Yamamoto, H. Salivary gland tumors in atomic bomb survivors, Hiroshima, Japan. I. Epidemiologic observations. *Cancer*, **38**, 2462–2468 (1976).
18. Takeichi, N., Hirose, F., Yamamoto, H., Ezaki, H., and Fujikura, T. Salivary gland tumors in atomic bomb survivors, Hiroshima, Japan. II. Pathologic study and supplementary epidemiologic observations. *Cancer*, **52**, 377–385 (1983).
19. Wood, J. W., Tamagaki, H., Neriishi, S., Sato, T., Sheldon, W. F., Archer, P. G., Hamilton, H. B., and Johnson, K. G. Thyroid carcinoma in atomic bomb survivors, Hiroshima and Nagasaki. *Am. J. Epidemiol.*, **89**, 4–14 (1969).

GANN Monograph on Cancer Research 32, 1986

MALIGNANT TUMORS IN ATOMIC BOMB SURVIVORS WITH SPECIAL REFERENCE TO THE PATHOLOGY OF STOMACH AND LUNG CANCER

Tsutomu YAMAMOTO,*[1] Issei NISHIMORI,*[2] Eiichi TAHARA,*[3] and Ichiro SEKINE*[2]

Department of Pathology, Radiation Effects Research Foundation,[1] *Department of Pathology, Atomic Disease Institute, Nagasaki University School of Medicine,*[2] *and Department of Pathology, Hiroshima University School of Medicine*[3]

A general review of stomach and lung cancer among atomic bomb (A-bomb) survivors is made classified by three time periods, 1945–60, 1960–75, and 1975–84. First is the period of "what is A-bomb disease?," during the second period the fixed population samples and the tentative 1965 radiation dose (T65D) estimates were established, and during the third period the tumor and tissue registries were operating and reassessment of radiation dose was underway. From review of stomach and lung cancer studies during the three time periods the following findings can be summarized: 1) the incidence of stomach and lung cancer among A-bomb survivors is related to radiation exposure dose, and the incidence of cancer increases at the usual ages when cancer appears, 2) cancer incidence is high among survivors who were exposed when young and the latent period is short, and 3) there is no specific histological type of radiation-induced cancer, but poorly differentiated types develop with a high frequency.

Of diseases suffered by atomic bomb (A-bomb) survivors in Hiroshima and Nagasaki, correlation with radiation dose has so far been observed only for malignant tumors, while for other diseases no such finding has been noted (*22*). Thus, it is important to focus interest on carcinogenesis due to A-bomb radiation not only for the welfare of survivors but also in ascertaining the mechanism of radio-carcinogenesis. This also means that the results of radiation-induced cancer in animal experiments may be an indication of similar effects in man. A-bomb survivors in Hiroshima and Nagasaki are the only large-scale population ever to experience whole-body exposure to a single dose of ionizing radiation.

In studying whether malignant tumors which developed in survivors are due to radiation or not, because radiation-induced cancers are not generally different from those otherwise present, it is necessary that epidemiological and statistical methods be used in comparative studies between findings of the exposed and nonexposed. Therefore, the following two requirements are essential: 1) definition of an exposed population, and 2) establishment of the radiation dose. Unfortunately, these two criteria have not yet been made even 39 years after the bombing. This has made it difficult to provide a clarifying

*[1] Hijiyama Park 5-2, Minami-ku, Hiroshima 732, Japan (山本　務).
*[2] Sakamoto-machi 12-4, Nagasaki 852, Japan (西森一正, 関根一郎).
*[3] Kasumi 1-2-3, Minami-ku, Hiroshima 734, Japan (田原栄一).

explanation for the so-called "A-bomb disease" which was used during the early years of studies on late A-bomb effects.

The study of cancer in survivors can be classified into the following three periods, the first period (1945–60), the second period (1960–75), and the third period (1975–84). During the first period, attention was focussed on the high incidence of leukemia and related disorders, but the study sample had not been well defined and all reports on exposure conditions were based on distance from ground zero, the tentative 1957 dose (T57D) estimates (*4*). During the second period, a fixed population consisting of approximately 100,000 subjects called the Life Span Study (LSS) sample was established in Hiroshima and Nagasaki by the Atomic Bomb Casualty Commission (ABCC) and the Japanese National Institute of Health (JNIH) (*18*). The T57D was revised and replaced with the tentative 1965 dose (T65D) (*26*) which was based on nuclear explosion tests in the US, and included individual exposure doses calculated with consideration given to shielding factors, whereas T57D was estimated from the air dose. The Unified Program was initiated based on three major programs, the Adult Health Study (AHS), the Pathology Study, and the LSS (*7*).

During the third period, the ABCC / Radiation Effects Research Foundation (RERF) Autopsy Study was phased out and Tumor Registries were established in Hiroshima and Nagasaki. Reassessment of radiation dose is also being made with new dose estimate expected in 1986. During the third period, attention began to be focussed on the occurrence of solid tumors other than leukemia.

Studies on the so-called "A-bomb disease" from the time of the A-bomb are extensive and diversified in scale and summarization will be attempted with the exception of certain periods which have been reported by others (*9*, *12*, *15*, *41*). We would like primarily to describe stomach cancer and lung cancer, a statistical summarization will be made first, after which reports will be made on each cancer.

The First Period

During the first period, studies were conducted by Obo (*33*), Beebe *et al.* (*5*), Ishida (*17*), Harada *et al.* (*14*), and Shimizu (*36*, *37*). In an attempt to resolve the question of "What is A-bomb disease?" Obo (*33*) classified 34,871 death certificates in Hiroshima from August 1945 to December 1959 by address, sex, age, and disease, and calculated the mortality rate for A-bomb survivors and the entire population of Hiroshima City. The mortality rate for survivors approximates the national average but is higher than the average for Hiroshima City and Prefecture. The shorter the distance from ground zero, the higher was the mortality. Obo stated that this was due to increased deaths from malignant neoplasms and that there were no other diseases of high frequency. Also in males, the mortality rates for stomach and lung cancer were higher than the national average.

Beebe *et al.* (*5*) reviewed the mortality rate for 1950–59 in the approximately 20,000 subjects of the AHS sample, a subsample of the LSS sample, and found that there was a relationship between radiation and leukemia, but not other causes of death.

In order to ascertain the state of development of malignant tumors in A-bomb survivors, the Hiroshima City Medical Association initiated a Tumor Registry program in Hiroshima City in May 1957 and in 1958 the Nagasaki City Medical Association started a registry in Nagasaki City. Ishida (*17*) and Harada *et al.* (*14*) compiled data for the 20 month period following initiation of the registry, in which it is shown that the morbidity rate of malignant neoplasms in survivors in 1957 and 1958 was higher closer to ground zero and the observed value within 1,000 m from ground zero was four times higher than the expected value. The ratio of the observed value to the expected value within 1,500 m from ground zero was 1.93 for stomach cancer and 4.31 for lung cancer.

Shimizu (*36*, *37*) in distinguishing A-bomb survivors from the nonexposed on the basis of holders of the A-bomb Survivor's Health Handbook in Hiroshima City attempted a comparison between the two groups from 1957–60 with the use of vital statistics death schedules, and observed that the number of deaths due to malignant tumors was large within 2,000 m from ground zero, but no difference was seen between recognized A-bomb patients and non-A-bomb handbook holders. Shigeto (*35*) in studying, by distance from ground zero and age, 83 stomach cancer cases and 44 lung cancer cases seen among 39,404 outpatients (36,514 in the Department of Internal Medicine and 2,890 in the Department of Surgery) at the Hiroshima A-bomb Hospital from September 1956 to August 1963, obtained similar findings.

In a review of 175 malignant tumor cases among 580 cases autopsied during 1953–65 at the Hiroshima Prefectural Hospital, Monzen and Kikuchi (*28*) studied the relation of radiation to malignant neoplasms. They observed that malignant tumors were more frequent in relatively aged survivors within 2,000 m from ground zero, but due to the small number of survivors the relationship of specific malignant tumors and histological characteristics to radiation could not be ascertained. In a review of malignant tumors among survivors during 20 years post-bomb, Nishimori *et al.* (*32*) conducted an analysis of 4,619 cases autopsied at the Nagasaki University School of Medicine and observed radiation effects by distance from ground zero, but could not demonstrate any specific findings related to radiation. Angevine and Jablon (*2*) and Angevine *et al.* (*3*) reviewed diseases peculiar to survivors among 2,450 cases autopsied at Hiroshima and Nagasaki during 1948–59, but could not detect malignant tumors related to radiation except for leukemia and thyroid cancer. They observed that studies on late A-bomb effects based on autopsy cases require statistical consideration and that in the accumulation of cases epidemiological bias in the autopsy cases should be excluded as much as possible. No statistical significance was demonstrated in the relation of radiation to stomach and lung cancer. Zeldis *et al.* (*48*) obtained results suggestive of radiation carcinogenesis, but they could not demonstrate any relation between cancer of specific organs and radiation dose.

The Second Period

Ciocco (*11*) studied cumulative mortality rates from October 1950 to August 1964 for members of the LSS sample who were over 50 years of age as of October 1950, by exposure distance (more than 1,400 m and less than 1,400 m from ground zero). In this study lung cancer mortality rate was higher in those within 1,400 m with a significant difference in males. Stomach cancer mortality tended to be higher in those exposed 1,400 m but no significant difference was observed. However, he noted that the relative risk was high for 1950–55. With the use of death certificates for 1958–64 in Nagasaki, Mitani and Kidera (*27*) studied 3,481 malignant tumor cases assigned International Classification of Diseases (ICD 7th edition) code 140–205 to determine the difference in malignant tumors, if any, between exposed and nonexposed persons. The mortality due to malignant tumors in exposed persons was two to three times higher than in the nonexposed and higher than the national corrected mortality rate. These findings, he noted, indicate that radiation effects should not be ignored, but he could not demonstrate any specific tumor which was elevated in incidence only in the exposed. The incidence of malignant tumors was observed to be high among young persons exposed at 20–30 years of age in both sexes.

Many reports have been made on the ABCC fixed population from the middle of the second period (1960–75) to the third period (1975–84). Beebe *et al.* (*6*) reported that of 2,539 ABCC autopsy cases for 1950–65 in Hiroshima and Nagasaki, 225 cases were exposed within 1,400 m from ground zero and that, applying the estimated radiation dose, a significant relationship between radiation dose and malignant tumors among the autopsy cases was observed for lung cancer and leukemia but the finding was only suggestive for bladder cancer and urinary tract cancer. In a mortality study (*8*), he described that the relationship was suggestive for respiratory cancer and not significant for digestive cancer. Maki *et al.* (*23*) using data of 66 lung cancer cases detected among the AHS sample during 1950–66 reported an elevated risk of lung cancer, thyroid cancer, and breast cancer.

In a mortality study for the period 1950–70, Jablon and Kato (*21*) reported mortality in the high dose radiation group to be larger than in the low dose group and the not-in-city at the time of the bomb (ATB) group. They indicated that specific malignant tumors related to radiation were leukemia and all malignant tumors, but the relation was weak for uterine cancer and stomach cancer. The lung cancer rate was significantly higher in the group exposed to 100 rad or more than those exposed to 0–9 rad, especially in males. Only 10 of the 1,600 deaths from stomach cancer were among those aged 0–9 ATB and, although the two cases that occurred in the 200 rad group were more than 15 times the expected rate, generally the relationship to radiation could not be defined. By period, a significant difference was observed for 1965–70 but not for other periods. Even when these mortality studies were extended to 1972 (*29*), the relationship between stomach cancer, which accounted for approximately 40% of deaths in the sample, and ionizing radiation could not be clarified. The autopsy rate in the LSS sample reached 40% at the early stage, but it decreased gradually to 25% by 1970. It was reported (*38*) that the relationship to radiation was not significant in any cancer except for certain types of cancer and the relationship cannot be demonstrated by autopsy diagnosis alone.

The Third Period

ABCC-RERF has periodically reported on mortality from malignant tumors among survivors on the basis of death certificates. According to the recent report of Kato and Schull (*22*) for the period up to 1982, the mortality due to leukemia has continued to decrease with a difference from that in the controls observed only in Hiroshima. Contrary to this, an increase was observed in mortality from solid tumors among the survivors. They observed that malignant tumors developed at a higher rate at the time corresponding to the spontaneous development period and that both relative risk and absolute risk tended to be higher the younger the age ATB. According to mortality studies, the malignant tumor sites at present found to be significantly related to radiation dose are lung, breast, stomach, esophagus, urinary tract, colon, and myeloma, and it was after 1980 that a relationship was observed between stomach cancer mortality and radiation.

Stomach Cancer

It has gradually become evident that epidemiological and statistical consideration is necessary in the study of carcinogenesis among A-bomb survivors, but during the early and middle stages of studies on the late radiation effects, attempts were made to determine the morphological specificity of stomach cancer among A-bomb survivors. Since stomach cancer is the most frequent malignant tumor among the Japanese, it is quite natural that attempts were made to elucidate such specificity.

Imai *et al.* (*16*) employed 24 surgical cases and 9 autopsy cases of stomach cancer among A-bomb survivors in Hiroshima and Nagasaki and, as controls, stomach cancer cases (62 autopsy cases and 132 surgical cases) examined at the Department of Pathology, Kyushu University, with the aim of ascertaining the frequency of stomach cancer among A-bomb survivors and changes in host (A-bomb survivors) response to cancer. In their study of stomach cancer they could not demonstrate any difference between the survivors and the controls for histological type, developmental patterns, and postoperative course. Murphy and Yasuda (*30*) studied age at onset, age at initial examination, survival period, site of development, histological type, *etc.*, using 533 surgical and autopsy cases of stomach cancer (187 exposed cases) observed at ABCC in Hiroshima from December 1948 to June 1957. In their study, those exposed within 2,500 m from ground zero were regarded as A-bomb survivors, but no difference in stomach cancer was observed between the exposed group and the nonexposed group. Since the late effects of radiation on tissue are nonspecific, it is considered difficult to determine the morphological difference between the exposed and the nonexposed. Autopsy cases are selective and in particular during the early stage the selection was not statistically random and thus autopsy cases of stomach cancer were not considered to be representative of all deaths due to stomach cancer. It was thus difficult to determine the difference only through the findings obtained from autopsy cases and clinical cases. In order to elucidate the difference, it is necessary to compare all cases of stomach cancer diagnosed in Hiroshima City and Nagasaki City including exposed cases.

Uraki (*39*) studied by sex, age, site of development, histological findings, metastasis, *etc.*, 639 cases of stomach cancer (111 exposed and 402 nonexposed) diagnosed from January 1955 to December 1964, at Hiroshima University but could not demonstrate any difference between the exposed and nonexposed cases. Yamamoto *et al.* (*43–45*) attempted a pathohistological study on a total of 535 cases consisting of mainly autopsy and some surgical cases of stomach cancer belonging to the fixed populations in Hiroshima and Nagasaki during 1961–68, 1961–69, and 1961–74. Though some of the histological types (*i.e.*, tubular medullary, scirrhous, and mucocellular) tended to be most frequent in the heavily exposed survivors, no relationship between stomach cancer as a whole and exposure dose could be observed. Nakamura (*31*) studied stomach cancer cases appearing on death certificates of those belonging to the fixed populations in Hiroshima and Nagasaki for the period 1950–73 with emphasis on the heavily exposed and observed that although the number of stomach cancer cases decreased with increase in exposure dose, the mortality rate in Hiroshima increased with dose to peak at 400–499 rad. The relationship with dose was weaker in Nagasaki than in Hiroshima, but the highest mortality rate was observed at 500 rad. Although the collection of death certificates with stomach cancer as cause of death is nearly 100% complete, the reliability of such diagnosis is limited. In case of stomach cancer in the LSS population during 1961–75, the confirmation rate

TABLE I. Incidence Rate and Relative Risk for Stomach Cancer by Radiation Dose, Hiroshima and Nagasaki, 1950–77

Item	T65D in rad					
	Total	0	1–49	50–99	100–199	200+
Stomach cancer	2,155	832	1,010	113	92	108
Annual incidence ($\times 10^5$)	113.7	111.2	111.9	112.5	123.2	155.6
Relative risk	—	1.0	1.0	1.0	1.1	1.6***
Person-years ($\times 10^3$)	1,895.6	748.3	902.7	100.5	74.7	69.4

*** $p<0.001$.

TABLE II. Relative Risk for Stomach Cancer by Age ATB and Radiation Dose

Age ATB	T65D in rad				
	0	1–49	50–99	100–199	200+
0–9	1.0	0.7	0.6	1.1	4.2*
10–19	1.0	1.3	2.2	2.6	3.8***
20–29	1.0	1.1	1.5	1.4	2.2***
30–39	1.0	0.9	0.8	1.0	1.4
40–49	1.0	1.0	0.9	1.1	1.4*
50+	1.0	1.1	1.0	1.0	1.1

* $p<0.05$, *** $p<0.001$.

(rate of clinical diagnosis confirmed by autopsy diagnosis) was 84.2% while the detection rate (rate of autopsy findings diagnosed clinically) was 75.6% (*46*). Attempts have been made to clinically detect stomach cancer patients by the cellular antibody technique, but since experimental techniques have not been established sufficiently, the relationship with dose has not yet been observed (*1*).

Matsuura *et al.* (*25*) recently collected as many stomach cancer cases in Hiroshima and Nagasaki as possible (2,155 cases diagnosed during 1950–77) and observed a statistically significant difference in the relationship with exposure dose. Confining themselves to the RERF LSS sample, they studied cases of clinical diagnosis, surgical cases, autopsy cases, and death certificate cases, and made full use of the tumor and tissue registries of the two cities. With regard to cases which had not been registered, they visited hospitals and clinics in the community in order to check the medical charts and collected 2,155 cases (1,720 in Hiroshima and 435 in Nagasaki) during 1955–77 and a histological review was made on 1,148 cases (53.3%). Table I shows the relative risk for stomach cancer cases by estimated exposure dose, using 1.0 as the relative risk for the 0 rad group. A significant ($p<0.001$) relationship with stomach cancer cases was observed in the 200+ rad group (Table I). When stomach cancer cases are divided by age ATB, the relative risk is significantly high in those less than 30 ATB group (Table II). The time period from radiation exposure to development of stomach cancer is shortest in the 50 and over age ATB group, but there is no difference by radiation dose in each age group. Although there is no specificity in the site of development of stomach cancer in A-bomb survivors, classification of histological types shows that well differentiated adenocarcinoma and poorly differentiated adenocarcinoma tend to be frequent in stomach cancer in those with low radiation dose and those with high radiation dose, respectively (Table III).

TABLE III. Histological Type of Stomach Cancer, by Radiation Dose

Histological type		T56D in rad				
		Total	0	1–99	100–199	200+
Well differentiated adenocarcinoma	Observed	451	189	241	7	14
	%	45.2	48.8	46.8	17.1	25.6
Poorly differentiated adenocarcinoma	Observed	346	122	183	19	22
	%	34.7	31.5	35.5	46.3	40.7
Mucinous adenocarcinoma	Observed	57	28	21	3	5
	%	5.7	7.2	4.1	7.3	9.3

It is noteworthy that this study has demonstrated a relationship between stomach cancer in A-bomb survivors and exposure dose, a high incidence of stomach cancer in those less than 30 ATB, and that poorly differentiated adenocarcinoma tended to be the most frequent type. Clinically, Ito *et al.* (*20*) detected 43 stomach cancer cases in a mass X-ray stomach examination of survivors conducted during 1971–82, and, making a comparison between 3,369 cases whose doses had been determined and 3,819 cases who were more than 3,000 m from ground zero, observed a relationship between stomach cancer and radiation dose in those exposed to 100+ rad.

Lung Cancer

Lung cancer has a high incidence ranking next in order to stomach cancer. Different from gastric cancer, it had been assumed from early days that lung cancer was associated with exposure to radiation. Comprehensive research began from the second period (1960–75) during which a comparatively large number of cases were accumulated.

Fujimoto (*13*) studied the relationship of sex, age, and histological type by distance from ground zero among 50 lung cancer cases (32 male and 18 female) who were treated as outpatients of the Hiroshima A-bomb Hospital from September 1956 through August 1965. He surmised that there was a correlationship between lung cancer and A-bomb radiation in that there were 26 cases within 2,000 m from ground zero, 9 cases beyond 2,000 m and 15 cases among the proximally exposed (within 1,500 m from ground zero). Yamada (*42*) reviewed 31 lung cancer cases autopsied at Hiroshima University during 1960–65 on the basis of sex, age, radiation exposure, histological type, *etc.* The age at death of all cases was over 50, and 23 cases (74.1%) were between age 60–79. There were 13 A-bomb survivors exposed at 1,000–2,000 m from ground zero of whom 9 had squamous cell carcinoma. Importance is being attached to internal irradiation through inhalation of residual radioactive substances as a cause of lung cancer among A-bomb survivors.

During 1950–60, a study of lung cancer in the LSS sample was conducted by Wanebo *et al.* (*40*). Lung cancer cases were collected through clinical diagnosis, the tumor registry, autopsy records, and death certificates, and it was strongly suggested that lung cancer incidence increased with radiation dose. Although lung cancer frequency among A-bomb survivors exposed to 90 rad was higher than the expected value, no difference in age at onset, histological type, and other epidemiological factors was observed with the control group. Mansur *et al.* (*24*) reviewed the same sample pathologically and conducted an analysis of 200 lung cancer cases autopsied during 1950–64, when the autopsy rate was high (about 40%). Although a significant increase in lung cancer incidence was observed among A-bomb survivors exposed to 128 rad or more, no histological type specific to lung cancer of A-bomb survivors has yet been found. Cihak *et al.* (*10*) carried out studies during 1961–70 after more autopsy cases had been accumulated. The relationship with radiation was determined for 204 (5.4%) lung cancer cases among 3,778 autopsy cases in the LSS sample and the histological type was classified according to the WHO Histological Classification. Lung cancer cases among A-bomb survivors exposed to 200 or more rad were compared with those exposed to less than 1 rad, and the former had an incidence twofold greater. Classification by histological type showed 39 cases (19.1%) were of small cell anaplastic type and there was a significant increase among the 200 or more rad group. The fact that lung cancer of small cell anaplastic type was found at high frequency among A-bomb survivors is a finding similar to a report at the time that many uranium mine workers also had the same type of lung cancer, and thus it was interpreted that this type was a specific type of radiation lung cancer.

It is important to exclude environmental factors other than radiation considered to cause malignant tumors in A-bomb survivors, but it is difficult to do so. Review of the relationship between lung cancer in A-bomb survivors and smoking should be made. Although Ishimaru *et al.* (*19*) attempted to elucidate the effects of radiation and smoking on lung cancer incidence by interviewing 198 pairs composed of confirmed lung cancer cases and their controls, a definite conclusion could not be made. Concerning this problem, Kato and Schull (*22*) state that radiation and smoking have an additive relation with lung cancer incidence, that is, each of them is independently associated with the incidence, but another report (*34*) indicates that it is impossible to identify whether the relationship is additive or multiplicative (the factors interacting with each other).

Yamamoto (*47*) collected 1,057 lung cancer cases from the LSS sample in Hiroshima and Nagasaki during 1950–80 through clinical diagnosis, surgical cases, autopsy diagnosis, death certificates, *etc.* He studied the relationship between lung cancer and exposure dose using the revised T65D, and also tried to classify histologically the 488 cases available for review. The incidence of lung cancer in the 100 or more rad exposed group in both Hiroshima and Nagasaki was significantly higher than that for their control 0 rad group and the same results were obtained from cases confirmed histologically (Table IV). This finding was observed in both males and females. Review by age ATB showed each age group with an exposure dose of 200 or more rad had a significant relationship with lung cancer incidence, and the incidence was highest among the 20–29 age group. For histological type, the incidence of small cell carcinoma in the 100 or more rad exposed

TABLE IV. Incidence of Lung Cancer by Radiation Dose, 1950–80 (Adjusted for City, Sex, and Age ATB)

Item	T65D in rad					
	Total	0(A)	1–49(B)	50–99(C)	100–199(D)	200+(E)
Observed	792	281	355	47	58	51
Expected		316.7	372.0	44.2	31.7	27.4
Person-years ($\times 10^3$)	2,046.7	807.6	975.2	108.4	80.7	74.8
Incidence rate ($\times 10^3$)		0.343	0.369	0.411	0.707	0.721
Relative risk		1.00	1.08	1.20	2.06	2.10

Test: A: D ***; A: E ***; Trend ***. *** $p<0.001$.

TABLE V. Histological Type of Lung Cancer by Radiation Dose (Adjusted for City, Sex, and Age ATB)

Histological type	Item	T65D in rad				
		Total	0(A)	1–49(B)	50–99(C)	100+(D)
Epidemoid carcinoma	Observed	105	41	42	8	15
	Relative risk		1.00	0.88	1.40	1.96
	Test		A: D*			
Small cell carcinoma	Observed	56	18	23	3	12
	Relative risk		1.00	1.08	1.16	3.43
	Test		A: D***			
Adenocarcinoma	Observed	140	46	66	7	21
	Relative risk		1.00	1.26		
	Test		A: D**			
Other	Observed	41	13	23	2	3
	Relative risk		1.00	1.61	1.20	1.35
	Test		A: D N.S.			

*** $p<0.001$, ** $p<0.01$, * $p<0.05$, N.S., not significant.

group was significantly higher than that in their control 0 rad group and other histological types (*i.e.*, adenocarcinoma and epidermoid carcinoma) were observed at a significantly higher rate in the 100 or more rad group (Table V). It should be noted that the three types of radiation-induced cancer, (small cell carcinoma, adenocarcinoma, and epidermoid carcinoma) which constitute the majority (about 80%) of all lung cancer histological types were also observed at a significantly higher rate in the 100 or more rad group. Compared with the other histological types, small cell carcinoma is of the poorly differentiated type, and thus it is understandable that the frequency of this type is high.

Outlook of Study on Cancer of A-bomb Survivors

On reviewing study results obtained heretofore, development in A-bomb survivors of malignant neoplasms excluding leukemia can be summarized as follows: 1) incidence of cancer of each organ increases with radiation dose at the predilection age for each cancer, 2) cancer incidence is higher among those exposed when young and their latent period is short, and 3) there is not a specific type of radiation induced cancer, but the poorly differentiated type develops with high frequency.

Since the period normally associated with increased incidence of most cancer is in the latter half of life, it is necessary to collect even cases with low incidence and continue to follow-up changes of malignant tumors in A-bomb survivors at regular intervals in order to study cancer incidence among those exposed when young. Although it has been considered heretofore that difference in the onset time of cancer in A-bomb survivors depends on organ sensitivity to radiation, involvement of some other factors is suggested in view of experience with gastric cancer and lung cancer cases. The relationship between lung cancer with complicated histological structure and radiation has been demonstrated since around 1965. However, it has only been since 1980 that the relationship between gastric cancer with simpler structure developing from the glandular epithelium and radiation has been confirmed. More factors might be involved in the development of lung cancer originating from the respiratory mucosa which is directly exposed to the air than in the development of gastric cancer from the gastric mucosa which is exposed only to stimulation by food. In histological classification, the poorly differentiated type is predominant for both stomach and lung cancer, so that involvement of radiation might be strong for the centrally located stem cells. According to the above results, it is considered that a new approach to study cancer in A-bomb survivors is needed.

REFERENCES

1. Akiyama, M., Yamakido, M., Otake, M., Belsky, J. L., Pastore, J. O., Kawamoto, S., Okawa, T., and Dock, D. S. Stomach cancer screening in the Adult Health Study population, Hiroshima 1971–72. RERF Tech. Rep. 7-77 (1977).
2. Angevine, D. M. and Jablon, S. Late radiation effects of neoplasia and other disease in Japan. *Ann. NY Acad. Sci.*, **114**, 823–831 (1964).
3. Angevine, D. M., Jablon, S., and Matsumoto, Y. S. ABCC-JNIH pathology studies, Hiroshima and Nagasaki. Report 1. October 1950-September 1962. *Natl. Cancer Inst. Monogr.*, **19**, 445–465 (1965).
4. Arakawa, E. T. Radiation dosimetry in Hiroshima and Nagasaki atomic bomb survivors. *New Engl. J. Med.*, **263**, 488–493 (1960).
5. Beebe, G. W., Ishida, M., and Jablon, S. Life Span Study, report number 1: Description of study, mortality in the medical subsample. October 1950–June 1958. ABCC Tech. Rep. 5-61 (1961).
6. Beebe, G. W., Yamamoto, T., Matsumoto, S., and Gould, S. E. ABCC-JNIH pathology studies, Hiroshima and Nagasaki, Report 2, October 1950-December 1965. ABCC Tech. Rep. 8-67 (1967).
7. Beebe, G. W. and Usagawa, M. The major ABCC samples. ABCC Tech. Rep. 12-68 (1968).
8. Beebe, G. W., Kato, H., and Land, C. E. Studies of the mortality of A-bomb survivors. 5. Mortality and radiation dose, 1950–1966. *Radiat. Res.*, **48**, 613–649 (1971).
9. Beebe, G. W. and Kato, H. Cancer other than leukemia in "A review of thirty years study of Hiroshima and Nagasaki atomic bomb survivors." *J. Radiat. Res.*, **16** (Suppl.), 97–107 (1975).
10. Cihak, R. W., Ishimaru, T., Steer, A., and Yamada, A. Lung cancer at autopsy in atomic bomb survivors and controls, Hiroshima and Nagasaki, 1961–70. 1. Autopsy findings and relation to radiation. *Cancer*, **33**, 1580–1588 (1974).
11. Ciocco, A. Mortality 1950–64 and disease and survivorship 1958–64, among sample members age 50 years or older, 1 October 1950. ABCC Tech. Rep. 18-65 (1965).
12. Finch, S. C. and Moriyama, I. The delayed effects of radiation exposure among atomic bomb survivors, Hiroshima and Nagasaki, 1945–79. A brief summary. RERF Tech. Rep. 16-78 (1978).
13. Fujimoto, Y. Bronchogenic carcinoma among A-bomb survivors in the Hiroshima Atomic Bomb Hospital. *Hiroshima Igaku*, **20** (Suppl.), 360–367 (1965) (in Japanese).
14. Harada, T., Ouchi, G., and Ishida, Y. Neoplasms among A-bomb survivors in Hiroshima: First report of Research Committee on Tumor Statistics. *Hiroshima Igaku*, **14**, 347–356 (1961) (in Japanese); *J. Natl. Cancer Inst.*, **25**, 1253–1264 (1960).
15. "Hiroshima and Nagasaki. The physical, medical, and social effects of the atomic bombings," ed. the Committee for Compilation of Materials on the Damage of the Atomic Bombs in Hiroshima and Nagasaki, pp. 161–203 (1979). Iwanami Shoten, Tokyo (in Japanese).
16. Imai, T., Enjoji, M., Tamai, K., Otsuka, H., and Kochi, J. Histological observation of stomach cancer among A-bomb survivors. *Nisshin Igaku*, **43**, 1–10 (1956) (in Japanese).
17. Ishida, Y. Epidemiological study of malignant tumors among A-bomb survivors in Hiroshima. *Hiroshima Igaku*, **12**, 1020–1022 (1959) (in Japanese).

18. Ishida, M. and Beebe, G. W. Research plan for joint JNIH-ABCC study of life span of A-bomb survivors. ABCC Tech. Rep. 4-59 (1959).
19. Ishimaru, T., Cihak, R. W., Land, C. E., Steer, A., and Yamada, A. Lung cancer at autopsy in atomic bomb survivors and controls, Hiroshima and Nagasaki 1961–70. 2. Smoking, occupation and A-bomb exposure. *Cancer*, **36**, 1723–1728 (1974).
20. Ito, C., Hasegawa, K., and Kumazawa, T. Investigation of stomach disease in atomic bomb survivors. The 5th report: prevalence of gastric cancer by dose in atomic bomb survivors. *Hiroshima Igaku*, **37**, 457–460 (1984) (in Japanese).
21. Jablon, S. and Kato, H. Studies of the mortality of A-bomb survivors, Report 6. Radiation dose and mortality 1950–1970. *Radiat. Res.*, **50**, 649–698 (1972).
22. Kato, H. and Schull, W. J. Life Span Study Report 9, Part 1. Cancer mortality among atomic bomb survivors, 1950–78. *Radiat. Res.*, **90**, 395–432 (1982).
23. Maki, H., Ishimaru, T., Kato, H., and Wakabayashi, T. Carcinogenesis in atomic bomb survivors. ABCC Tech. Rep. 24-68 (1968).
24. Mansur, C. G., Keehn, R. J., Hiramoto, T., and Will, D. W. Lung cancer among atomic bomb survivors, Hiroshima-Nagasaki 1950–64. ABCC Tech. Rep. 19-68.
25. Matsuura, H., Yamamoto, T., Sekine, I., Ochi, Y., and Otake, M. Pathological and epidemiologic study of gastric cancer in atomic bomb survivors, Hiroshima and Nagasaki, 1950–77. *J. Radiat. Res.*, **25**, 111–129 (1984).
26. Milton, R. C. and Shohoji, T. Tentative 1965 dose (T65D) estimation for A-bomb survivors, Hiroshima and Nagasaki. ABCC Tech. Rep. 1-68 (1968).
27. Mitani, Y. and Kidera, A. A survey on the mortality rate of the exposed people in relation to the malignant disease. *Hiroshima Igaku*, **20** (Suppl.), 406–413 (1967) (in Japanese).
28. Monzen, T. and Kikuchi, H. Relation of malignant neoplasms and atomic bomb radiation in autopsy cases at Hiroshima Prefectural Hospital. *Hiroshima Igaku*, **20** (Suppl.), 394–403 (1965) (in Japanese).
29. Moriyama, I. M., and Kato, H. JNIH-ABCC Life Span Study, Report 7. Mortality experience of A-bomb survivors 1970–1972, 1950–1970. ABCC Tech. Rep. 15-73 (1973).
30. Murphy, E. S., and Yasuda, A. Carcinoma of the stomach in Hiroshima, Japan. *Am. J. Pathol.*, **34**, 531–542 (1958).
31. Nakamura, K. Stomach cancer in atomic bomb survivors, 1950–73. RERF Tech. Rep. 8-77 (1977).
32. Nishimori, K., Shigematsu, A., Hayakawa, A., Matsui, M., Tsuda, N., Hayashi, I., Sugiura, H., Matsuoka, S., and Noguchi, T. Malignant neoplasms of autopsy cases in Nagasaki. *Hiroshima Igaku*, **20** (Suppl.), 414–416 (1965) (in Japanese).
33. Obo, G. Statistical study on the causes of death occurring among atomic bomb survivors. *Hiroshima Igaku*, **14**, 323–334 (1961) (in Japanese).
34. Prentice, R. K., Yoshimoto, Y., and Mason, M. W. Cigarette smoking and radiation exposure in relation to cancer mortality, Hiroshima and Nagasaki. *J. Natl. Cancer Inst.*, **170**, 611–612 (1982).
35. Shigeto, F. Annual report of Hiroshima Atomic Bomb Hospital. (The 5th Meeting of Late Effects Research Group). *Hiroshima Igaku*, **17**, 634–645 (1964) (in Japanese).
36. Shimizu, K. A tendency of cancer death in Hiroshima City. Part 1. On the comparison of survivors health cards between issued and nonissued persons. *Hiroshima Igaku*, **13**, 885–889 (1960) (in Japanese).
37. Shimizu, K. Statistical study on A-bomb exposed cancer patients in Hiroshima. *Hiroshima Igaku*, **18**, 229–312 (1965) (in Japanese).
38. Steer, A., Moriyama, I. M., and Shimizu, K. ABCC-JNIH pathology studies, Report 3. The autopsy program and the Life Span Study. ABCC Tech. Rep. 16-73 (1973).
39. Uraki, J. Malignant neoplasms of the digestive organs, especially of gastric cancer. *Hiroshima Igaku*, **20** (Suppl.), 378–381 (1967) (in Japanese).

40. Wanebo, C. K., Johnson, K. G., Sato, K., and Thorslund, T. W. Lung cancer following atomic radiation. *Am. Rev. Respir. Dis.*, **88**, 778–787 (1968).
41. Watanabe, S. Cancer and leukemia developing among atomic bomb survivors. *In* "Handbuck der allgemeinen pathologie," ed. by W. Altmann, F. Buchner, H. Cottier, E. Grundmann, G. Holle, E. Lettere, W. Masshoff, H. Meesen, F. Roulet, G. Seifert, and G. Siebert, pp. 523–530 (1974). Springer-Verlag, Berlin, Heidelberg, New York.
42. Yamada, A. Summary of malignant tumors—Pathomorphological review of lung cancer observed among A-bomb survivors in Hiroshima. *Hiroshima Igaku*, **20** (Suppl.), 368–377 (1967) (in Japanese).
43. Yamamoto, T., Kato, H., Ishida, K., Tahara, E., and McGregor, D. H. Gastric carcinoma in a fixed population, Hiroshima-Nagasaki 1961–1968. *Gann*, **61**, 473–483 (1970).
44. Yamamoto, T. and Kato, H. Two major histological types of gastric carcinoma among the field population of Hiroshima and Nagasaki. *Gann*, **62**, 381–387 (1971).
45. Yamamoto, T. and Shimizu, Y. Relation of radiation to gastric carcinoma observed in autopsy cases in a fixed population, Hiroshima and Nagasaki 1961–74. *J. Radiat. Res.*, **19**, 213–227 (1978).
46. Yamamoto, T., Moriyama, I., Asano, M., and Guralnick, L. The autopsy program and the life span study, Report 4 January 1961–December 1975. *J. Hiroshima Med. Assoc.*, **32**, 267–276 (1979).
47. Yamamoto, T. Lung carcinoma of A-bomb survivors in Hiroshima and Nagasaki 1950–80. The 24th Lung Cancer Society of Japan, Hiroshima, Oct. 1983. (Abstr., in Japanese).
48. Zeldis, L. J., Jablon, S., and Ishida, M. Current status of ABCC-JNIH studies of carcinogenesis in Hiroshima and Nagasaki. *Ann. NY Acad. Sci.*, **114**, 225–240 (1964).

GANN Monograph on Cancer Research 32, 1986

COLORECTAL CANCER AMONG ATOMIC BOMB SURVIVORS

Hirofumi NAKATSUKA*[1] and Haruo EZAKI*[2]
Second Department of Surgery, Hiroshima University School of Medicine[1] *and Department of Clinical Studies, Radiation Effects Research Foundation*[2]

Studies on autopsied and surgical cases of colorectal cancer in Hiroshima and Nagasaki atomic bomb (A-bomb) survivors have not shown a relationship to radiation.

In a recent epidemiologic study made on a fixed population at the Radiation Effects Research Foundation (RERF), the risk of colon cancer was found to increase significantly with increasing radiation dose in both Hiroshima and Nagasaki, and also in both males and females. The dose effect for the cities and sexes combined was especially pronounced for cancer of the sigmoid colon. The effect of radiation was found to vary by age at the time of the bomb (ATB) and the effect was remarkable among those under age 20 ATB. The risk of rectal cancer was not found to increase significantly with radiation and the distribution of histological types for cancer of either the colon or rectum was unrelated to radiation dose.

The effect of A-bomb exposure on the postoperative survival rate for colorectal cancer patients was studied. No difference by radiation dose could be demonstrated.

In Japan, the incidence of colorectal cancer, and of colon cancer in particular, has been increasing. Therefore, close attention should be paid to changes occurring in A-bomb survivors.

Experimental evidence suggests that intestinal tumors, especially malignant tumors, can be induced in mice by whole-body irradiation (*23*, *27*). In man, the development of colorectal cancer following pelvic irradiation for benign disorders or cancer of the cervix and uterus has been reported (*3*, *5*, *24*). Also, a study of patients treated for ankylosing spondylitis by radiation showed an excess of deaths from cancer of the large intestine (*4*).

In atomic bomb (A-bomb) survivors, diarrhea and bloody stools were observed as clinical symptoms of acute radiation sickness, and inflammation and ulcerative lesions of the mucosa of the intestinal tract were found histopathologically (*15*). Therefore, it is suspected that the intestinal tract was subject to considerable damage by ionizing radiation.

According to a recent report (*12*) on the RERF Life Span Study (LSS) sample, a radiation effect has been observed for colon cancer but not for rectal cancer. However, only a few reports have been made concerning the occurrence of malignant tumors of the large bowel in A-bomb survivors.

*[1] Kasumi 1-2-3, Minami-ku, Hiroshima 734, Japan (中塚博文).
*[2] Hijiyama Park 5-2, Minami-ku, Hiroshima 732, Japan (江崎治夫).

In this paper, the reports made to date on colorectal cancer in A-bomb survivors are summarized, the effect of A-bomb radiation on the occurrence of colorectal cancer is reviewed, and data on the postoperative survival rate for colorectal cancer patients are included.

Colorectal Cancer in Autopsied Cases

Liebow *et al.* (*15*) reported that hemorrhage and ulceration occurred very frequently in the gastrointestinal tract of patients who died between the third and sixth weeks after the bombings. Further, ulcerative lesions of the intestine, especially of the colon, occurred often in those who died after the sixth week. However, reports have rarely been made on autopsied cases in relation to the occurrence of malignant tumors in the intestinal tract.

Yamamoto and Kato (*31*) reported on 94 cases of malignant tumor of the intestinal tract found among the autopsied cases in the Atomic Bomb Casualty Commission (ABCC) and the Japanese National Institute of Health (JNIH) fixed population during the period 1948–70. In that report, which dealt with the tumor site, age distribution, and histological type, no relationship with radiation dose was observed.

Colorectal Cancer in Surgical Cases

Regarding surgical cases of colorectal cancer in A-bomb survivors of Hiroshima, 32 cases of colon cancer were reported by Sato *et al.* (*25*) and 25 cases of rectal cancer by Miyoshi *et al.* (*19*). According to these reports, colorectal cancer in survivors was characterized by the predominance of cases in advanced age, relatively advanced stages, and a high proportion of local infiltration which rendered radical resection impossible. Recently, Nakatsuka *et al.* (*21*) analyzed the postoperative survival of 81 A-bomb survivors of Hiroshima who had undergone surgery for colorectal cancer during 1958–82; they found no statistically significant difference in the survival rate between these cases and those in 198 nonexposed persons in the same period.

Azuma *et al.* (*1*) conducted a clinical study on 119 cases of colorectal cancer in Nagasaki survivors and reported a high rate of second primary cancer in these survivors.

Because the number of cases was small and there were problems with respect to the selection of control groups, these reports have not been able to demonstrate definitively the features of colorectal cancer in the population of survivors.

Colorectal Cancer in the RERF LSS Sample

In 1950, ABCC-JNIH established a fixed sample of approximately 100,000 subjects consisting of A-bomb survivors and their controls in Hiroshima and Nagasaki (*10*), and RERF is continuing a long-term follow-up study of this sample. Colorectal cancer in this sample will be discussed.

According to Beebe *et al.* (*2*), an analysis of mortality for the period 1950–74 did not demonstrate any obvious radiation effect in either colon cancer or rectal cancer. A significant relationship between colon cancer and radiation dose was found only among Hiroshima females. Tumor Registry data for the period 1959–70 showed a statistically significant increasing trend in incidence of colon cancer with increasing dose in both

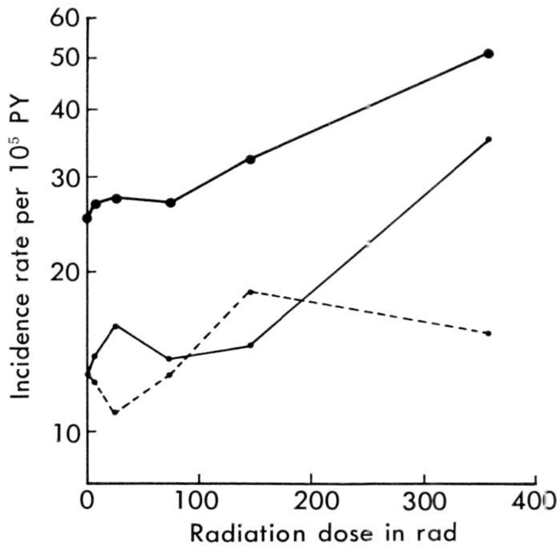

FIG. 1. Colorectal cancer incidence rate by radiation dose and organ, Hiroshima and Nagasaki, 1950–80 (adjusted for age ATB, sex, and city). ●—●, colorectal*** (551 cases); •—•, colon*** (286 cases); •---•, rectum[NS] (test for linear trend; NS, $p>0.10$; *** $p<0.001$).

Hiroshima ($p<0.02$) and Nagasaki ($p<0.05$). However, the incompleteness of the Tumor Registry data and possible bias in identification of cases leave problems that need to be resolved. Subsequently, Kato and Schull (*12*) extended the study period to 1950–78, and reported a significant association between radiation dose and colon cancer mortality. An association between radiation dose and colon cancer incidence was also suggested by the analysis of Wakabayashi *et al.* (*28*) who used data from the Nagasaki Tumor Registry for the period 1959–78. However, in no study reported so far has there been observed any relationship between rectal cancer and A-bomb radiation.

Motivated by the results described above, Nakatsuka *et al.* (*22*) conducted a review of the relationship between exposure dose (tentative 1965 dose revised (T65DR)) (*13*, *18*) and incidence of colorectal cancer. This study included a clinicopathological reexamination of cases in the LSS Extended Sample who were diagnosed as colorectal cancer based on the autopsy and surgical specimens of ABCC-RERF, Hiroshima and Nagasaki Tumor and Tissue Registry data, and death certificates for 1950–80.

According to this study, the incidence of colon cancer among A-bomb survivors increased significantly with radiation dose ($p<0.001$), but that of rectal cancer did not ($p>0.10$) (Fig. 1).

1. City and sex

These data showed a statistically significant increasing trend in the incidence of colon cancer with increasing dose in both Hiroshima ($p<0.001$) and Nagasaki ($p<0.05$) (Fig. 2). A dose response was also found for males ($p<0.01$) and for females ($p<0.001$) (Fig. 3).

2. Age at the time of the bomb (ATB)

The relative risk of colon cancer in the 100 or more rad dose group as compared to the 0 rad group differed by age ATB, being especially large for those exposed at age less than 20 (Table I).

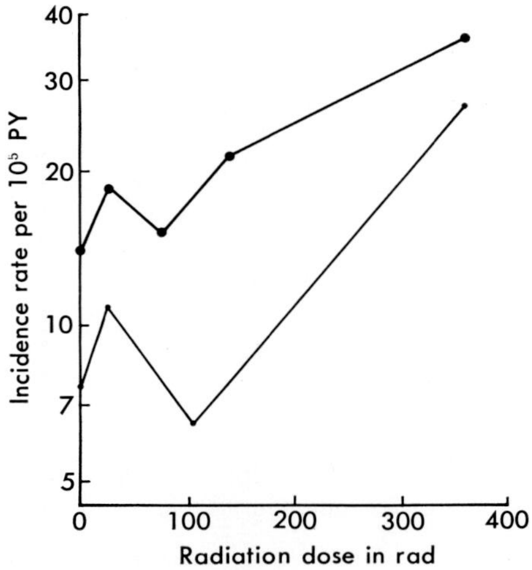

FIG. 2. Colon cancer incidence rate by radiation dose and city (adjusted for age ATB and sex). ●—●, Hiroshima*** (239 cases); •—•, Nagasaki* (47 cases) (test for linear trend; * $p<0.05$; *** $p<0.001$).

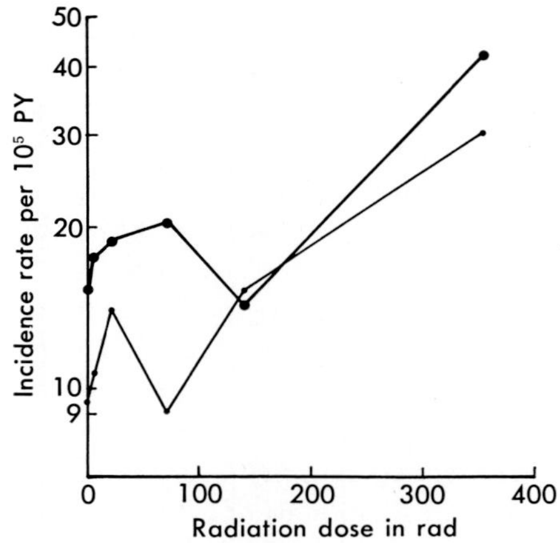

FIG. 3. Colon cancer incidence rate by radiation dose and sex (adjusted for age ATB and city). ●—●, male** (145 cases); •—•, female** (141 cases) (test for linear trend; ** $p<0.01$).

TABLE I. Relative Risk of Colon Cancer Incidence by Age ATB and Period (100+ *vs.* 0 rad)

Period	Age ATB in years					
	Total	20	20–29	30–39	40–49	50+
Total	2.0**	4.5**	2.1	1.7	1.8$^{Sug.}$	1.3
	(99,33)	(6,7)	(8,4)	(31,9)	(32,9)	(22,4)
1950–64	1.3	—	—	2.1	0	1.2
	(16,3)	(0,0)	(0,1)	(4,1)	(5,0)	(7,1)
1965–80	2.1**	5.3**	1.5	1.7	2.1*	1.5
	(83,30)	(6,7)	(8,3)	(27,8)	(27,9)	(15,3)

Numbers in parentheses are colon cancer cases in the 0 rad and 100+ rad groups, respectively.
Two-sample Mantel-Haenszel test: Suggestive, $p<0.10$; * $p<0.05$; ** $p<0.01$.

3. Primary site of colon cancer

A radiation effect was observed for cancer originating in each of the following sites: cecum plus ascending colon ($p<0.01$), transverse plus descending colon ($p<0.05$), and sigmoid colon ($p<0.001$). Among these sites, the dose-response effect was most remarkable in the sigmoid colon (Fig. 4).

4. Histopathological type

Cancer was classified by histological type according to the General Rules for Clinical and Pathological Studies on Cancer of Colon, Rectum, and Anus (*11*). Neither

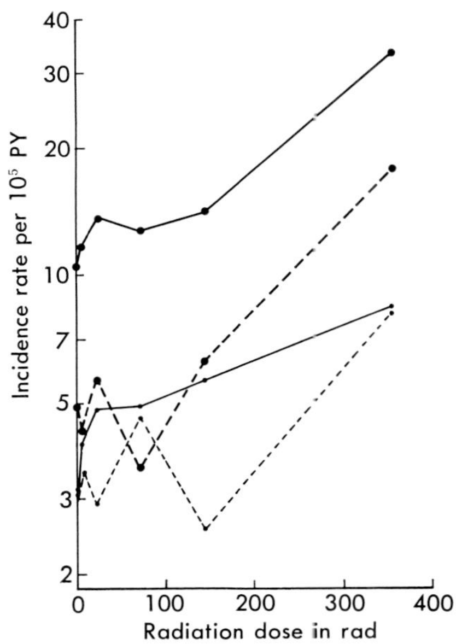

FIG. 4. Colon cancer incidence rate by radiation dose and site-confirmed cases (adjusted for age ATB, sex, and city). ●—●, colon*** (251 cases); ●---●, sigmoid*** (111 cases); •—•, cecum+ascending** (76 cases); •---•, transverse+descending* (64 cases) (test for linear trend; * $p<0.05$; ** $p<0.01$; *** $p<0.001$).

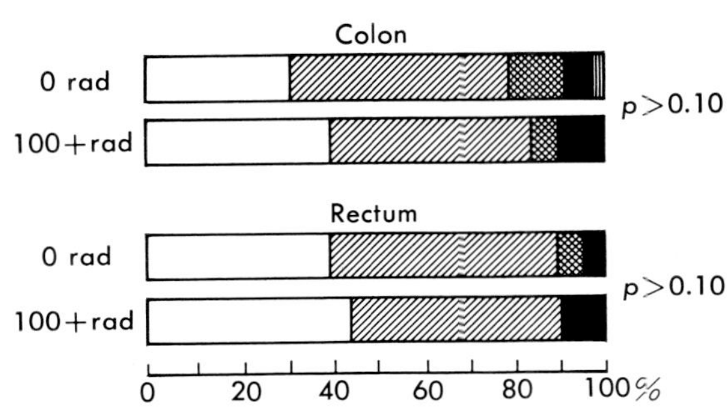

FIG. 5. Distribution of histological type of colorectal cancer by radiation dose. □, well differentiated adenocarcinoma; ▨, moderately differentiated adenocarcinoma; ▩, poorly differentiated adenocarcinoma; ■, mucinous carcinoma+signet ring cell carcinoma; ||||, other.

colon nor rectal cancer showed a significant difference in distribution of histopathological type between the 0 rad group and the 100 or more rad group (Fig. 5).

Survival of Colorectal Cancer Patients after Surgery

A study was made on the effects of A-bomb exposure on the postoperative survival rate for colorectal cancer patients (*20*).

Of the 730 cases, surgery was performed on 545 cases, of whom 148 cases who died within one month after surgery or whose records were missing were excluded from the analysis (Table II). Figure 6 shows the cumulative survival rates by type of surgery and cancer site.

For colon cancer the survival rate was highest for curative resection followed by noncurative resection and without resection. For rectum cancer, the survival rate of curative resection was the highest, followed by noncurative resection and without resection, the latter two being at almost the same level. The difference in the survival rates was found to be significant by the Mantel-Cox test (*16*).

TABLE II. Number of Operated Cases by Type of Operation and Cancer Site

Type of operation	Site			
	Total	Colon	Rectum	Unknown
Total	397	218	178	1
Curative resection[a]	238	134	103	1
Noncurative resection[a]	85	58	27	—
Without resection	62	22	40	—
Polypectomy	6	2	4	—
Unknown	6	2	4	—

Excluding operative deaths and cases whose stage of cancer, age, sex, and date of surgery are unknown.
[a] General Rules for Clinical and Pathological Studies on Cancer of Colon, Rectum, and Anus," 2nd ed., Japanese Research Society for Cancer of Colon and Rectum, 1980.

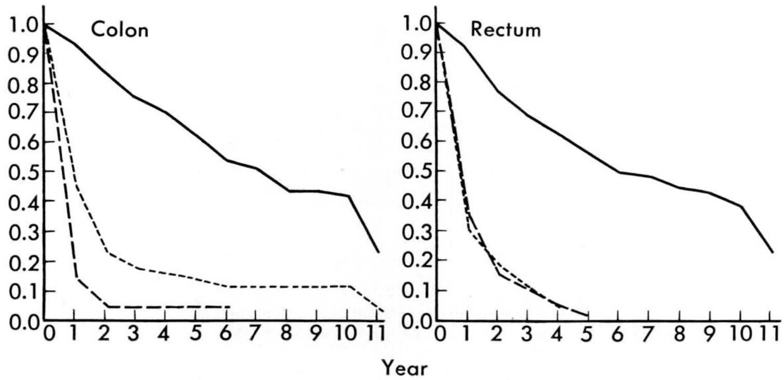

FIG. 6. Cumulative survival rate by type of operation. Colon: ——, curative resection (n=134); ----, non curative resection (n=58); — —, without resection (n=22); Mantel-Cox test, $p<0.001$. Rectum: ——, curative resection (n=103); ----, non curative resection (n=27); — —, without resection (n=40); Mantel-Cox test, $p<0.001$.

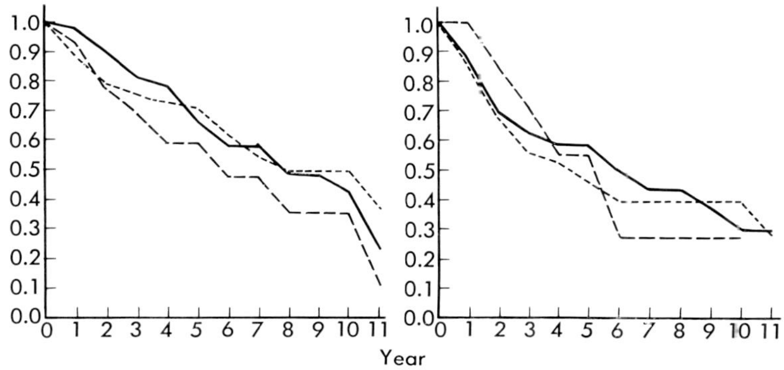

FIG. 7. Cumulative survival rate by radiation dose. Colon: ——, 0 ($n=39$); ----, 1–99 ($n=52$); — —, 100+ ($n=13$); Mantel-Cox test, $p>0.10$. Rectum; ——, 0 ($n=33$); ----, 1–99 ($n=34$); — —, 100+ ($n=7$); Mantel-Cox test, $p>0.10$.

The relationship between survival rate and radiation dose was examined for only cases of curative resection. Cases whose exposure dose was unknown and those who were not in the city ATB were excluded (Fig. 7). The survival rate of colon cancer cases tended to be slightly lower in the 100 or more rad group than in the other two groups. For rectum cancer, the survival rate for the 100 or more rad group was better than for the other groups during the early postoperative period, but the long-term survival rate of this group was found to be slightly lower. However, comparison of the survival curves of these groups by the Mantel-Cox test demonstrated no statistically significant difference.

As there are many factors which affect the postoperative survival rates, it is necessary to examine the effects of other factors in order to determine the effect of radiation. The potential factors are age at the time of operation, period of operation, sex, stage of cancer, and histopathological grade of cancer (Fig. 8). No difference could be observed by age, period of operation, and histopathological grade of cancer. By sex, the survival rates for both colon and rectum cancer cases were significantly higher in females. The survival rate of colon cancer cases was observed to be higher in Group A of Dukes' classification than in Groups B and C, but the difference was not statistically significant. The survival rate of rectum cancer cases was significantly higher in the order of A, B, and C.

It is necessary to take these factors into account in order to determine the effect of A-bomb exposure on the postoperative survival rate. For this purpose, classification into many groups with the same factors is necessary, but such classification makes the number of cases in each cell so small that comparison is not possible. By using Cox's proportional hazard model, which enables comparison of survival curves while taking into account the effects of many factors simultaneously, the regression coefficient of each group was examined, but no difference by radiation dose could be demonstrated in the postoperative survival rate for either colon or rectum cancer.

DISCUSSION

The occurrence of intestinal cancer due to radiation exposure has been confirmed by animal experiments (*8*, *23*, *27*). Malignant tumors have been noted to develop in humans

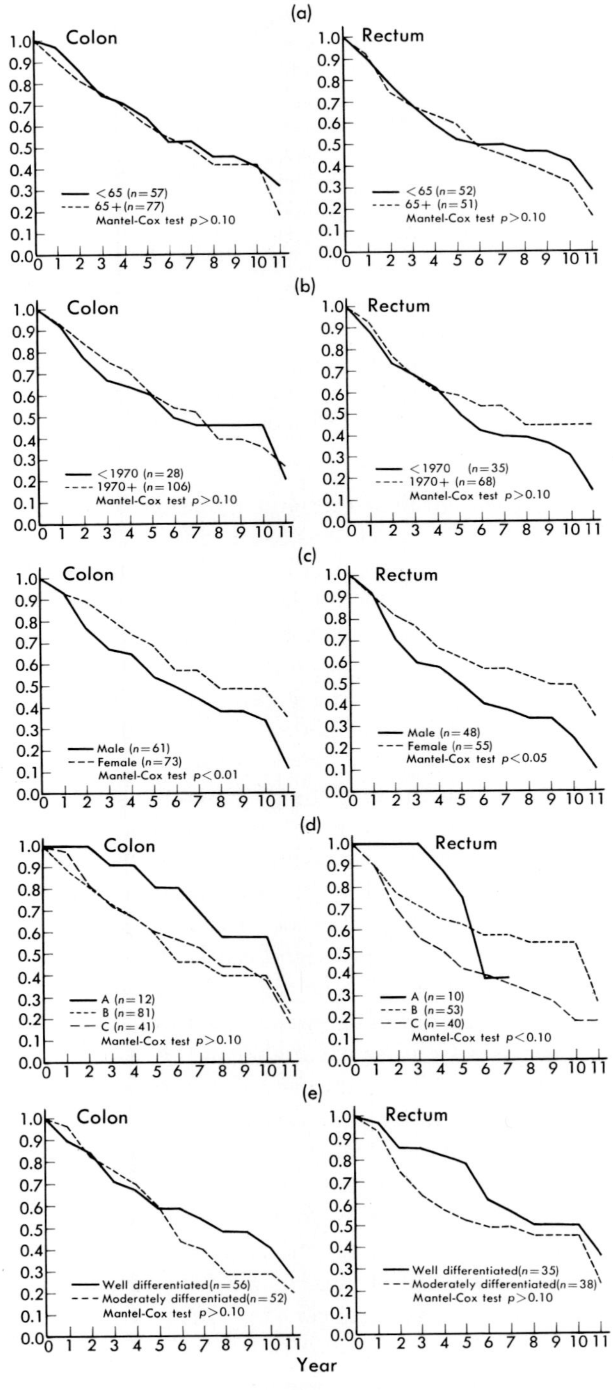

FIG. 8. Survival rate by age at operation (a), period at operation (b), sex (c), stage of cancer (Dukes' classification) (d), and histopathological grade (e).

following radiation therapy for lesions of the uterus or ovary (*3*, *24*): tumors were found to originate in the part of the large bowel that lay in the irradiation field.

However, among epidemiological studies made so far on man, there have been few reports of a definite effect of radiation in the genesis of colorectal cancer.

In RERF studies on the LSS population, a significant relationship with ionizing radiation has been observed for colon cancer, but not for rectal cancer, and the radiation effect on the colon was remarkable for sigmoid colon. Such a difference in A-bomb radiation effect by site for colorectal cancer is of great interest, since it has been reported from epidemiological studies (*7*, *29*, *30*) that the colon is more susceptible than the rectum to carcinogenic effects of exogenous factors such as diet, and that this tendency is remarkable in the sigmoid colon.

In a comparison between Hiroshima and Nagasaki, a difference was observed in the incidence of leukemia (*9*), perhaps due to the difference of radiation quality. However, no obvious difference in the colon cancer dose-response relationship has been observed between the two cities (*22*). This problem should be studied further since the radiation dose estimates are currently being reassessed.

The effect of age ATB on the occurrence of malignant tumors is being studied in detail with regard to hormone-dependent tumors such as breast cancer (*26*) and thyroid cancer (*6*). Matsuura *et al.* (*17*) reported on stomach cancer, which, among digestive organ cancer, showed a remarkable elevation in incidence in those under age 30 ATB. On the other hand, Nakatsuka *et al.* (*22*) reported that they found an elevation in the incidence of colon cancer in those exposed to 100 or more rad who were under age 20 ATB, and that this group needs to be followed very carefully as it is now reaching the age when colon cancer is prone to develop.

The distribution of histological types shows no difference between the radiation dose groups. Castro *et al.* (*3*) reported that the percentage of mucinous carcinoma is high in cases exposed to medical radiation; however, the cases they reported were exposed to high partial-body doses of several thousand rad as therapy for cervical or uterine cancer. The A-bomb survivors, in contrast, are a general population exposed to an average of 27.2 rad (*12*).

The present report centers around studies which are based on a fixed population of A-bomb survivors, and which concern the effect of ionizing radiation on the occurrence of colorectal cancer. In recent years in Japan colorectal cancer, and colon cancer in particular, has shown a gradually increasing trend (*14*, *29*) possibly due to westernization of diet and an increasing number of people of advanced age. Thus it remains imperative to pay attention to changes occurring in atomic bomb survivors.

REFERENCES

1. Azuma, K., Yamashita, I., Noda, S., Sakaeda, K., and Noguchi, K. Colorectal cancer in atomic bomb survivors in the Japanese Red Cross Nagasaki A-bomb Hospital. *Jpn. J. Gastroenterol. Surg.*, **14**, 869 (1981) (in Japanese).
2. Beebe, G. W., Kato, H., and Land, C. E. Life Span Study Report 8. Mortality experience of atomic bomb survivors, 1950–74. RERF Tech. Rep. 1-77 (1977).
3. Castro, E. B., Rosen, P. P., and Quan, S.H.Q. Carcinoma of large intestine in patients irradiated for carcinoma of cervix and uterus. *Cancer*, **31**, 45–52 (1973).
4. Court Brown, W. M. and Doll, R. Mortality from cancer and other causes after radiotherapy for ankylosing spondylitis. *Br. Med. J.*, **2**, 1327–1332 (1965).

5. Doll, R. and Smith, P. G. The long term effects of x-irradiation in patients treated for metropathia heamorrhagica. *Br. J. Radiol.*, **41**, 362–368 (1968).
6. Ezaki, H. Thyroid cancer occurring in Hiroshima atomic bomb survivors (1958–79). *J. Jpn. Pract. Surg. Soc.*, **44**, 1127–1137 (1983) (in Japanese).
7. Haenszel, W. and Correa, P. Cancer of the colon and rectum and adenomatous polyps; A review of epidemiologic findings. *Cancer*, **28**, 14–24 (1971).
8. Hirose, F., Fukazawa, K., Watanabe, H., Terada, Y., Fujii, I., and Otsuka, S. Induction of rectal carcinoma in mice by local x-irradiation. *Gann*, **68**, 669–680 (1977).
9. Ishimaru, T., Hoshino, T., Ichimaru, M., Okada, H., Tomiyasu, T., Tsuchimoto, T., and Yamamoto, T. Leukemia in atomic bomb survivors, Hiroshima and Nagasaki, 1 October 1950–30 September 1966. *Radiat. Res.*, **45**, 216–233 (1971).
10. Jablon, S., Ishida, M., and Beebe, G. W. JNIH-ABCC Life Span Study, Report 2 Motality in selection 1 and 2, October 1950—September 1959. *Radiat. Res.*, **21**, 423–445 (1964) (ABCC Tech. Rep. 1-63).
11. Japanese Research Society for Cancer of Colon and Rectum (ed). "General Rules for Clinical and Pathological Studies on Cancer of Colon, Rectum and Anus," The 2nd ed. (1980) Kanehara Publishing Company, Tokyo (in Japanese).
12. Kato, H. and Schull, W. J. Studies of mortality of A-bomb survivors. 7. Mortality, 1950–78: Part 1. Cancer mortality. *Radiat. Res.*, **90**, 395–432 (1982) (RERF Tech. Rep. 12-80).
13. Kerr, G. D. and Solomon, D. L. The epicenter of the Nagasaki weapon: A reanalysis of available data with recommended values. Oak Ridge National Laboratory, ORNL-TM-5139, U.S.A. (1979).
14. Lee, J.A.H. Recent trends of large bowel cancer in Japan compared to United States and England and Wales. *Int. J. Epidemiol.*, **5**, 187–194 (1976).
15. Liebow, A. A., Warren, S., and DeCoursey, E. Pathology of atomic bomb casualties. *Am. J. Pathol.*, **25**, 853–1029 (1949).
16. Mantel, N. Evaluation of survival data and the new rank order statistics arising in its consideration. *Cancer Chemother., Rep.*, **50**, 163–170 (1966).
17. Matsuura, H., Yamamoto, T., Sekine, I., Ochi, Y., and Otake, M. Pathological and epidemiologic study of gastric cancer in atomic bomb survivors, Hiroshima and Nagasaki, 1959–77. *Radiat. Res.*, **25**, 111–129 (1984).
18. Milton, R. C. and Shohoji, T. Tentative 1965 radiation dose estimation for atomic bomb survivors, Hiroshima and Nagasaki. ABCC Tech. Rep. 1-68 (1968).
19. Miyoshi, Y., Seto, Y., Morinaga, K., Yukata, H., Hirose, S., Sasaki, K., and Ogawa, Y. Surgical studies of rectal cancer at the Hiroshima Atomic Bomb Hospital for 10 years. *J. Hiroshima Med. Assoc.*, **33**, 313–315 (1980) (in Japanese).
20. Nakatsuka, H., Ezaki, H., and Shimizu, Y. Survival rate of colorectal cancer patients after surgery. In preparation.
21. Nakatsuka, H., Tamura, T., Nishiki, M., Kodama, M., and Ezaki, H. Review of colorectal cancer cases in atomic bomb survivors. *Abstr. Gen. Meet. Jpn. Pract. Surg. Soc.*, **44**, 486 (1983) (in Japanese).
22. Nakatsuka, H., Yamamoto, T., Shimizu, Y., Takahashi, M., Ezaki, H., Tahara, E., Sekine, I., Shimoyama, T., Mochinaga, N., Tomita, M., and Tsuchiya, R. Colorectal cancer among atomic bomb survivors in Hiroshima and Nagasaki (1950–80). Collection of lectures of 25th Late A-bomb Radiation Effect Research Meeting. *Nagasaki Med. J.*, **59**, 473–480 (1984) (in Japanese).
23. Nowell, P. C., Cole, L. J., and Ellis, M. E. Induction of intestinal carcinoma in the mouse by whole-body fast-neutron irradiation. *Cancer Res.*, **16**, 873–876 (1956).
24. Sandler, R. S. and Sandler, D. P. Radiation-induced cancer of the colon and rectum: Assessing the risk. *Gastroenterology*, **84**, 51–57 (1983).
25. Sato, M., Yo, S., Sasao, T., Sasaki, K., and Ogawa, Y. Surgical studies of colon cancer at

the Hiroshima Atomic Bomb Hospital for 10 years. *Nagasaki Med. J.*, **53**, 398–403 (1978) (in Japanese).

26. Tokunaga, M., Norman, J., Asano, M., Tokuoka, S., Ezaki, H., Nishimori, I., and Tsuji Y. Malignant breast tumors among atomic bomb survivors, Hiroshima and Nagasaki, 1950–74. *J. Natl. Cancer Inst.*, **62**, 1347–1359 (1979) (RERF Tech. Rep. 17-77).
27. Upton, A. C., Kimball, A. W., Furth, J., Christenbery, K. W., and Benedict, W. H. Some delayed effects of atomic bomb radiation in mice. *Cancer Res.*, **20**, 1–60 (1960).
28. Wakabayashi, T., Kato, H., Ikeda, T., and Schull, W. Life Span Study Report 9, part 3, Tumor Registry data, Nagasaki 1959–78. RERF Tech. Rep. 6-81 (1981).
29. Watanabe, Y., Kawamoto, K., Kajiwara, Y., Akasaka, Y., and Kawai, K. Epidemiological study on cancer of the large intestine in Japan (1) Fundamental analysis from mortality of the large intestine in Japan. *J. Jpn. Soc. Colo-proctol.*, **36**, 607–614 (1983) (in Japanese).
30. Wynder, E. L. The epidemiology of large bowel cancer. *Cancer Res.*, **35**, 3388–3394 (1975).
31. Yamamoto, T., and Kato, H. Malignant tumors of the intestines found in a fixed population of Hiroshima. *Proc. Jpn. Cancer Assoc.*, **30**, 112 (1971).

GANN Monograph on Cancer Research 32, 1986

BREAST CANCER IN ATOMIC BOMB SURVIVORS

Masayoshi TOKUNAGA,[*1,*2] Shoji TOKUOKA,[*3] and Charles E. LAND[*4]

Department of Pathology, Kagoshima Municipal Hospital,[*1] *Department of Pathology and Department of Epidemiology and Statistics, Radiation Effects Research Foundation,*[*2] *Second Department of Pathology, Faculty of Medicine, Hiroshima University,*[*3] *and Radiation Epidemiology Branch, National Cancer Institute, NIH*[*4]

Thirty eight years after the atomic bombings, studies of the Radiation Effects Research Foundation (RERF) on the extended Life Span Study (LSS) sample have continued to provide important information on radiation carcinogenesis. The third breast cancer survey among this sample revealed 564 cases during the period 1950–80, of which 412 were reviewed microscopically. The following statements reflect the conclusions from the current investigation; 1) the relationship between radiation dose and breast cancer incidence was consistent with linearity and did not differ markedly between the Hiroshima and Nagasaki survivors, 2) a dose-related breast cancer risk was observed among women who were in their first decade of life at the time of exposure, 3) the relative risk of radiation-induced breast cancer decreased with increasing age at exposure, 4) the pattern over time of age-specific breast cancer incidence is similar for exposed and control women (that is, exposed women have more breast cancer than control women but the excess risk closely follows normal risk as expressed by age-specific population rates), and 5) radiation-induced breast cancer appears to be morphologically similar to other breast cancer.

There is general agreement that ionizing radiation is one of the best understood and most thoroughly studied environmental carcinogens and that female breast cancer may be the best understood site of radiation-induced cancer in humans.

In 1965, Mackenzie (*13*) reported an increased risk of breast cancer for women who received repeated fluoroscopy during pneumothorax treatment for tuberculosis in a Nova Scotia sanatorium. At that time, he found 13 cases of breast cancer in 271 patients subjected to repeated chest fluoroscopy as compared with only one case which developed in 570 patients who were not fluoroscoped. This study group was later extended by Myrden and Hiltz (*17*).

Boice and Monson (*5*) studied 1,047 women treated in Massachusetts tuberculosis sanatoria by pneumothorax who received an average of 102 chest fluoroscopies during 1935–54, and a control group of 717 nonexposed tuberculosis patients. Many of the patients had been treated as teenagers, in contrast to the Nova Scotia series in which

*1 Kajiya-cho 20-17, Kagoshima 892 and *2 Hijiyama Park 5-2, Minami-ku, Hiroshima 730, Japan (徳永正義).

*3 Kasumi 1-2-3, Minami-ku, Hiroshima 734, Japan (徳岡昭治).

*4 Landow Building, Room 3A22, Bethesda, Maryland 20892, U.S.A.

patients were appreciably older when treated. Individual dosimetry yielded an estimated average breast tissue dose of 150 rad in 100 exposures, averaging 1.5 rad per exposure. Breast cancer incidence was high among the exposed (41 observed *vs.* 23.5 expected according to population rates), and the excess was proportional to dose. The excess risk was estimated as 6.2 breast cancer cases per million women per year per rad. The minimal appearance time for radiogenic breast cancer was estimated to be 10 to 15 years, while the risk extended for as long as 40 years after exposure. The Massachusetts data were interpreted as suggesting that early adult life is a time when the breast is particularly susceptible to cancer induction, that proliferating tissue may be sensitive to irradiation, and that multiple low-dose exposures cumulated over many years may be as effective in inducing breast cancer as less fractionated, or even single, exposures (*2, 5*).

Radiation induced breast cancer was observed among women with histories of X-ray therapy for acute postpartum mastitis by the studies of Mettler *et al.* (*15*) and Shore *et al.* (*18*). Shore *et al.* (*18*) found 36 (6.3%) breast cancer cases in 571 women treated with X-rays for acute postpartum mastitis compared with 32 (3.2%) in 933 nonirradiated siblings and patients treated by other means. The mean cumulative dose to both breasts was 247 rad, and the overall excess risk of breast cancer was about 8–10 cases per million women per year per rad. Women over age 30 years at radiation treatment had as great an excess risk of breast cancer as did younger women. A linear dose response was observed, and the relatively minor fractionation of exposure (1–5 fractions) did not appear to reduce carcinogenic action.

Baral *et al.* (*1*) reported a study of women given radiation therapy for benign breast disorders in Sweden, and found young women to be at greatest radiation risk; generally risk decreased with age at exposure.

In addition to these breast cancer studies among medically exposed populations, continuing follow-up studies of breast cancer incidence among female survivors of the Hiroshima and Nagasaki atomic bomb (A-bomb) explosions provided important knowledge about radiation breast carcinogenesis. In 1967, Wanebo *et al.* (*24*) studied 31 cases of breast cancer (27 with histological diagnoses) occurring among examined members of the Atomic Bomb Casualty Commission (ABCC) Adult Health Study (AHS) sample of A-bomb survivors in Hiroshima and Nagasaki for the period 1958–66. Of the 18 histologically verified cases occurring among exposed women examined at least once during the period 1958–66, and for whom dose estimates could be made, 50% had dose estimates of 90 rad or more as compared to only 24% expected by chance alone.

In 1974, McGregor *et al.* (*14*) studied breast cancer incidence among members of the much larger ABCC Life Span Study (LSS) sample for the period 1950–69. In this study, 231 breast cancer cases were identified among 63,275 female A-bomb survivors and nonexposed controls and 187 were among survivors for whom dose estimates were available. The estimated absolute risk per rad was 1.9 excess cases per 10^6 person-years at risk. The data suggested that the breast tissue of adolescent females, as compared to older women, was especially sensitive to the effects of ionizing radiation.

The similarity observed by McGregor *et al.* (*14*) between the two cities was interesting partly because baseline (that is, nonradiogenic) breast cancer rates in Nagasaki have historically been only about half those in Hiroshima, but mainly because the radiation from the Hiroshima bomb was for a long time believed to contain a substantial neutron component absent in the radiation from the Nagasaki bomb. Neutrons generally are more damaging than gamma rays, and indeed, excess risk for cancer other than breast cancer has tended to be greater in Hiroshima than in Nagasaki. Approximate equality of the excess risk per unit dose between the two cities was interpreted as suggesting approximate equivalence of gamma ray and neutron radiation for the induction of breast cancer. More recent dosimetric studies suggest that the quality of the radiation received from the two bombs was not so different after all; reassessment of dosimetry is now underway, and for the present it is difficult to evaluate this aspect of the breast cancer data from Hiroshima and Nagasaki.

The second incidence study among the extended LSS sample was performed by Tokunaga *et al.* (*22*) and increased the number of cases to 360 during 1950–74. This incidence survey found similar dose-incidence relationships, both consistent with linearity, in Hiroshima and Nagasaki. Age at exposure was an important biological modifier of risk, with the greatest relative and absolute increase occurring among those 10 to 19 years at the time of the bomb (ATB). No excess risk was observed among those exposed under age 10 ATB, although it was recognized that these women might not yet be old enough for a risk to be detected. A rather peculiar relationship was observed among those 40 to 49 ATB in that no radiation related risk was detected, and as dose increased, the incidence of breast cancer actually decreased.

Summary of Findings Prior to the Third LSS Survey

The nearly simultaneous publications in 1979 of epidemiological studies of breast cancer risk in three different irradiated populations, the Boice-Monson study (*5*) of Massachusetts tuberculosis patients with multiple chest fluoroscopies, the Shore *et al.* (*18*) survey of patients given X-ray therapy for benign breast disease in Rochester, New York, and the second ABCC-RERF (1950–74) study (*22*) based on the extended LSS sample of A-bomb survivors in Hiroshima and Nagasaki prompted a reanalysis in parallel of the basic data from all three studies (*4*, *10*). The central feature of this reanalysis was that, in so far as possible, the data were identically subdivided by age at exposure, and risk was observed for closely similar periods following exposure. For similar exposure ages, risk estimates obtained by linear regression of risk on radiation dose were closely similar for the three data sets, despite differences in underlying population rates, fractionation of exposure, and the extent to which irradiation extended to parts of the body other than the breast (Fig. 1). These differences were substantial, including a five-fold difference between Japanese and American population rates, a single exposure among the A-bomb survivors *vs.* 1–19 fractions among the Rochester patients and 100 or more fractions among the Massachusetts tuberculosis patients, and whole-body A-bomb exposure *vs.* chest irradiation from fluoroscopy *vs.* therapeutic X-ray limited to one or two breasts. For all three data sets the observed dose response appeared linear, a finding that is consistent with the lack of a dose fractionation effect. Other important characteristics of the three data sets were, first, that excess risk did not appear until ages of normally appreciable breast cancer risk, regardless of age at exposure, and that after it appeared the temporal patterns of excess and background risk were closely similar. Second, at ages of normally appreciable risk, the excess following exposure at ages 10–19 was markedly higher than that following exposure at older age.

The observation that multiple low-dose exposures did not produce significantly less cancer per unit dose than less highly fractionated exposures suggests that radiation damage is cumulative and that highly fractionated X-irradiation may be as effective in

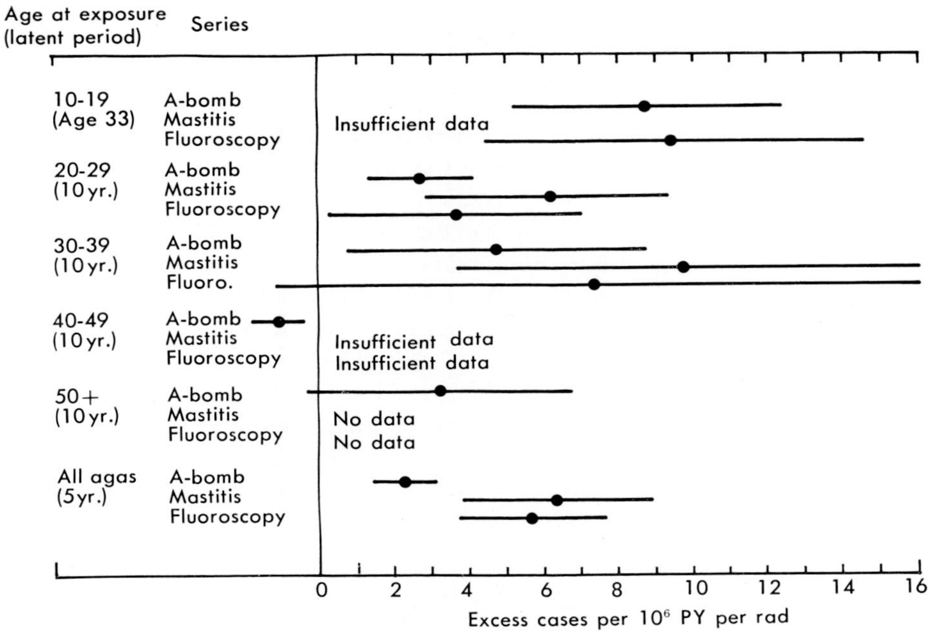

FIG. 1. Excess breast cancer risk per rad with 90% confidence intervals: parallel and analysis of three exposed populations.

inducing breast cancer as single or less fractionated exposures. The interpretation of these results is of particular public health importance, since the radiation of usual medical examination, cancer screening, or therapy is received from repeated exposure to low dose.

The Third LSS Follow-up Survey

As in the two earlier surveys of breast cancer incidence in the LSS extended sample (*14*, *22*), an attempt was made to ascertain all diagnoses of breast cancer obtainable from resources available locally in Hiroshima and Nagasaki. The most wide-ranging of these resources is the system by which death certificate diagnoses routinely are made available to RERF from death certificates filed anywhere in Japan for members of the LSS sample. All death certificates for 1950–80 with breast cancer listed as either the underlying cause, a complication, or a contributing condition were included in the initial ascertainment. Information was collected from the series of indexed cases in the RERF autopsy program, the RERF collection of surgical specimens, the Tumor Registries maintained since 1959 and the Tissue Registries maintained since 1971 by the City and Prefectural Medical Associations of Hiroshima and Nagasaki, the records of the medical schools of Hiroshima and Nagasaki Universities, and records of more than 50 hospitals in both cities.

A total of 564 breast cancer cases was identified for the period 1950–80 among the 63,300 women in the extended LSS sample, which includes nearly all residents of Hiroshima and Nagasaki in 1950 who had been exposed within 2,500 m from ground zero, 15,400 nonexposed women who migrated or returned to the cities after August 1945, and an age-matched sample of women exposed between 2,500–10,000 m from ground zero.

1. *Histological classification*

Of the total of 564 female cases finally selected, 412 were accepted on the basis of pathology review. Of these, 301 cases were included in a review by a binational panel of pathologists from Japan and the United States on the basis of an incomplete ascertainment of cases through 1978 (*23*). The distribution of histological types in exposed and nonexposed groups is presented in Table I for the 412 cancer cases reviewed histologically by the investigators. According to contingency table analysis there was no evidence that the histological type is related to city, age ATB, age at diagnosis, calender time, radiation dose, or any combination of these factors. In particular, there was no tendency for one or more histological types or subtypes to characterize radiation-induced breast cancer. Although there have been no reported pathological studies of breast cancer among medically exposed populations, the present results provide strong evidence that radiation induced breast cancer appears to be morphologically similar to other breast cancer. One interpretation of these results is that the histological type of breast cancer is influenced by other factors but not by whether or not radiation is one initiator.

2. *Linear dose response*

The most important finding of the studies to date is that of linearity of the dose response for radiation-induced breast cancer, together with the similar pattern of risk for the two cities (Fig. 2). Linear regressions of age-standardized rates on total (gamma ray plus neutron) tentative 1965 dose (T65D) to breast tissue gave estimates of 4.0 ± 0.7 and 3.0 ± 0.7 excess cases per million women per year per rad for Hiroshima and Nagasaki,

TABLE I. Distribution of Histological Type of Breast Cancer by Dose

Histological type	T65D in rad							
	NIC[c]	0–9	10–49	50–99	100–199	200+	Unknown	Total
Noninvasive[a]	4	6	—	1	—	2	—	13
Invasive								
a. Ductal								
0. CSF[b]	8	17	2	4	3	10	1	45
1. Papillotubular	5	7	4	—	0	2	2	20
2. Medullary tubular	14	24	9	7	2	7	4	67
3. Scirrhous	31	91	27	4	16	14	3	186
b. Predominant ductal component	7	21	9	2	3	3	—	45
c. Lobular	—	1	1	1	2	—	—	5
d. Mucinous	—	7	—	—	—	2	—	9
e. Medullary	1	3	—	—	—	—	—	4
f. Tubular	—	—	0	2	—	—	—	2
g. Secretory	—	1	—	—	—	1	—	2
h. Apocrine	—	1	—	—	—	—	—	1
i. Carcinoma with metaplasia	—	—	—	—	—	1	—	1
j. Paget's Disease								
0. *In situ* only	1	1	2	—	—	—	—	4
1. With invasive carcinoma	—	0	2	—	1	—	—	3
k. Other	2	3	—	—	—	—	—	5
Total	73	183	56	21	27	42	10	412

[a] All noninvasive carcinomas were intraductal; there were no lobular carcinomas *in situ*.

[b] Cannot subclassify further.

[c] Not in the city.

ovary) were detected in 61 (8.4%) of 721 patients an average of 16 years after they received radiation therapy. The number of cancer cases detected was higher than expected, based on a survey of clinical diagnoses and death certificates, in the same district during the same period. The highest incidence rate of postradiation cancer (11.8-fold greater than expected) was seen in the vagina, and the lowest (1.7-fold) in the cervix. The incidence rate of postradiation cancer of the ovary was 3.1-fold higher than expected. The findings of Palmer and Spratt (*17*) contradict the hypothesis (*6*, *18*) that carcinogenesis following radiation exposure is primarily attributable not to the effect of radiation, but to the endocrine abnormality concealed within the background of the primary lesion against which the radiation therapy was employed.

Many studies dealing with carcinogenesis following radiation therapy for benign lesions or malignant tumors in the gynecological organs have appeared (*1*, *3*, *7*, *16*, *22*, *24*). For example, Boice *et al.* (*3*) recently reported that the relative risk of ovarian cancer developing after high dose radiation therapy for cancer of the uterine cervix in patients of North American and European countries was significantly increased 20 years after exposure.

Court Brown and Doll (*5*) found increased ovarian cancer mortality in a sample of 14,554 patients, including 2,393 females, who had been treated with X-rays for ankylosing spondylitis. This increased mortality was due not only to leukemia and aplastic anemia but also to cancer of organs in proximity to the sites of heavy exposure (the mortality due to the latter was increased as much as 2-fold 6 years after the initial exposure). In a similar study in which the sample was restricted solely to patients who had received a single course of X-ray therapy, the mortality due to cancer in organs near the irradiated sites was 60% higher than the general cancer mortality of respective organs (*21*).

A number of deaths in older women among Marshall Islanders who had been exposed to whole-body gamma rays from fallout, have been attributed to cancer of the genital organs (*4*). An increased incidence of leukemia, as well as cancer in various organs, has been found in the atomic bomb (A-bomb) survivors of Hiroshima and Nagasaki, Japan, but reports concerned only with ovarian cancer in female survivors are few. Two cases, one of a 27-year-old female who suffered from granulosa-theca cell tumor of the ovary 8 years after exposure in Hiroshima, and the other of a 30-year-old female who suffered from serous cystadenocarcinoma of the ovary 12 years after exposure at the same city, have been described (*11*, *19*). Based on a study of death certificates in Hiroshima during the 5 year period commencing in 1951, a report (*23*) indicated that the morbidity of both breast and ovarian cancer was increased in exposed females. Another analysis, from tumor cases registered in 1957–58, showed a significant excess of ovarian cancer in females who were exposed within 1,500 m from ground zero in Hiroshima (*9*).

A mortality study based on death certificates among females in the Radiation Effects Research Foundation (RERF) Life Span Study (LSS) extended sample in Hiroshima and Nagasaki during 1950–82 has shown a substantially high correlation between the incidence of ovarian cancer and exposure dose (*10*). Recently, Tokuoka *et al.* (*26*) conducted a pathological and epidemiological study of ovarian tumors in the same LSS sample, and ascertained 194 malignant and 106 benign tumors of the ovary, which had occurred during the 31-year period from 1950–80. All available data sources (RERF autopsy and surgical pathology records, medical schools, hospitals, tumor and tissue registries of both cities, and death certificates) were employed for ascertainment of tumor cases.

TABLE I. Age-adjusted Incidence Rate (per 1,000 person-years) of Ovarian Cancer by Exposure Dose

Method of ascertainment	Item	Total	T65 dose in rad							Test[b]
			0	1–9	10–99	100–199	200+	Unknown	NIC[a]	
Total	Cases	194	74	27	31	10	9	2	41	
	Person-years	1,834,383	662,111	348,705	304,586	46,876	43,058	33,646	395,400	
	Age-adjusted incidence rate (/ 1,000)	0.106	0.111	0.078	0.078	0.237	0.242	0.081	0.104	$p<0.01$
Histologically reviewed cases	Cases	128	51	17	19	5	7	1	28	
	Person-years	1,834,383	662,111	348,705	304,586	46,876	43,058	33,646	395,400	
	Age-adjusted incidence rate (/ 1,000)	0.070	0.077	0.049	0.060	0.117	0.183	0.040	0.069	$p<0.01$

[a] Not in city ATB.

[b] Statistical test for linear increase with dose (excluding unknown and NIC).

Of the 194 cases of ovarian cancer, 128 (66%) were reviewed microscopically by the authors of this study. The remaining 66 cases included 19 histologically diagnosed cases from which tissue materials were not available for study, 28 cases in which surgical removal of the tumor was performed under the clinical diagnosis of ovarian cancer, and 19 cases with a clinical diagnosis of ovarian cancer in either the clinical record or in the death certificate.

Of the 194 cases 79 (40.7%) were exposed to 1 rad or more of radiation (*15*); these were grouped by estimated exposure dose as shown in Table I. Note that 36 of the 58 cases (62.1%) who received an exposure dose of 1–99 rad were reviewed microscopically. In comparison, the microscopical confirmation rate in 19 cases exposed to 100 or more rad was 63.2% (12/19); the microscopical confirmation rates in the 0 rad group and the nonexposed group were 68.9% (51/74) and 68.3% (28/41), respectively. There were no statistically significant differences in the histological confirmation rates among these groups. On this basis, examination for an increased incidence of ovarian cancer among exposed compared to nonexposed individuals, and for any relationship between incidence and magnitude of dose exposure among exposed individuals, can be made either with all ascertained cancer cases, or solely with microscopically reviewed cases.

Excluding the 41 nonexposed and 2 dose-unknown individuals among the 194 cases, the age-adjusted incidence rate of ovarian cancer per year per 1,000 persons by exposure dose among the remaining 151 exposed cases showed a statistically significant ($p<0.01$) linear increase with increased exposure dose (Table I and Fig. 1). This linear dose response remained significant ($p<0.01$) when only the 128 microscopically reviewed exposed cases were considered. The linear dose response was not apparent in the first half of the study period (1950–64), but was present ($p<0.01$) in the latter half (1965–80), both in microscopically reviewed cases (Fig. 2) as well as in all cases.

The relative risk of ovarian cancer incidence in the 100 or more rad group compared to the 0 rad group, by age at the time of the bomb (ATB), was highest in the youngest age group, less than 20 ATB, and was lower in those exposed at older ages (Table II).

Since the LSS began in October 1950, the postexposure latent period for tumor development can be estimated by adding five years and two months, that is, the period

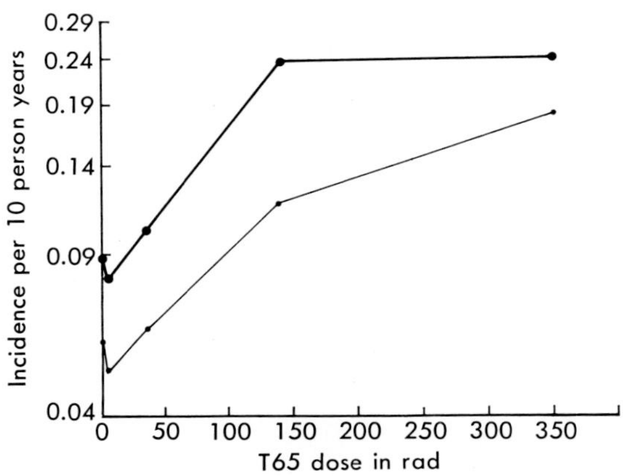

FIG. 1. Incidence of ovarian cancer by exposure dose and method of ascertainment, Hiroshima and Nagasaki 1950–80. ●, all cases ($p<0.01$); •, microscopically reviewed cases ($p<0.01$).

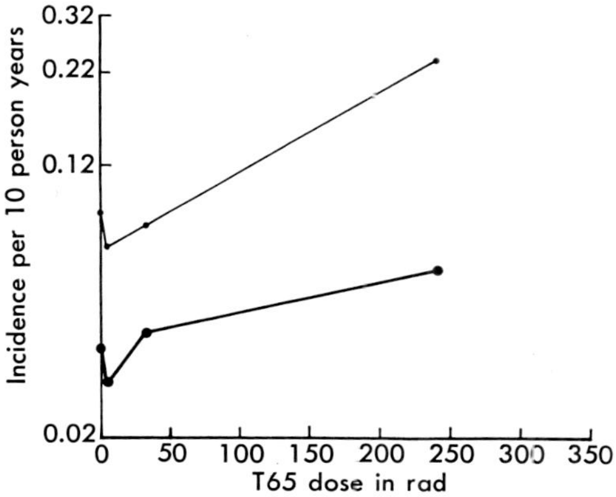

FIG. 2. Incidence of ovarian cancer by exposure dose and study period, Hiroshima and Nagasaki (microscopically reviewed cases). ●, 1950–64 ($p>0.10$); •, 1965–80 ($p<0.01$).

TABLE II. Relative Risk (100+ rad *vs.* 0 rad) of Ovarian Cancer Incidence by Age ATB

Method of ascertainment	Total	Age ATB in years				
		<20	20–29	30–39	40–49	50+
Total	2.2	5.0	2.1	1.5	1.5	0.95
	(74,19)	(9,7)	(14,5)	(18,3)	(18,3)	(15,1)
Histologically	1.9	4.4	2.5	1.1	1.9	—
reviewed cases	(51,12)	(6,4)	(10,4)	(16,2)	(9,2)	(10,0)

The numbers in parentheses are the number of cases in the 0 rad and 100+ rad groups, respectively.

TABLE III. Mean Time in Years from 1950 (Beginning of Follow-up) to Onset of Ovarian Cancer—All Cases

Age ATB in years	Total	T65 dose in rad				
		0	1–99	100+	Unknown	NIC[a]
Total	17.6±0.6	17.8±1.0	17.4±1.1	19.3±1.5	19.2±11.1	16.5±1.1
<20	21.8±1.2	26.2±0.9	25.3±1.1	21.3±1.3		17.1±2.8
20–39	18.9±0.9	20.2±1.3	17.5±1.9	19.6±3.1	19.2±11.1	17.8±1.7
40+	14.5±0.8	13.2±1.4	15.7±1.5	15.3±2.8		14.9±1.5

[a] Not in city ATB.

of time from exposure to the time of study commencement, to the average time for tumor development determined from the LSS (Table III).

In this regard, it was found that the latent period was not affected by the magnitude of exposure dose, but that it was inversely related to age ATB in all dose groups. For example, in the 100 or more rad group, the latent period was 15.3±2.8 years (the shortest) in the age group 40 and over ATB, 19.6±3.1 years in the age group 20–29 ATB, and 21.3±1.3 years (the longest) in the age group less than 20 ATB. This suggests that, as with breast cancer (*25*), ovarian cancer in A-bomb survivors does not develop until the host reaches an age normally associated with increased incidence, irrespective of either

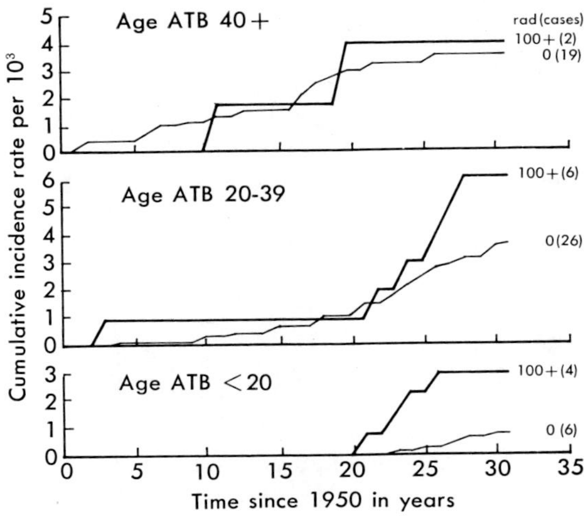

FIG. 3. Cumulative incidence rate (per 1,000) by exposure dose and ATB, Hiroshima and Nagasaki (microscopically reviewed cases).

age ATB or exposure dose; moreover, the latent period until tumor development is unrelated to exposure dose. Note, however, that in the age group less than 20 ATB, the mean latent period in the 100 or more rad exposure group was 21.3±1.3 years, which appears to be significantly shorter than 26.2±0.9 years in the 0 rad group; although the number of cases is quite small. The age group less than 20 ATB includes many individuals who had not reached the cancer age at the time of this study; this will necessitate further follow-up studies.

The cumulative incidence rate of ovarian cancer per 1,000 persons for the total 31 year period (1950–80) is shown in Fig. 3, stratified by the two exposure groups (100 or more rad *vs.* 0 rad) and three age ATB groups. An excess in the incidence rate for the 100 or more rad group *vs.* that for the 0 rad group was observed 10–15 years after 1950 (*i.e.*, 15–20 years after exposure) for the age 40 or more ATB group. For the age less than 20 ATB group, an excess in the incidence rate apparently comes later, around 25 years after exposure.

The finding also suggests that the minimum latent period for radiation induced ovarian cancer would be around 15–20 years, and the latent period is inversely related to age ATB.

The distribution of the 128 microscopically reviewed cases of ovarian cancer by histological type is shown in Table IV. Of the 128 cases 121 (94.5%) were carcinomas that belong to the WHO (*20*) category "Common Epithelial Tumors" (I). Of the remaining seven cases, four were granulosa cell tumors of "Sex Cord Stromal Tumors" category (II), two were teratomas associated with malignant transformation, and one was carcinoid, belonging to the "Germ Cell Tumors" category (IV).

The histological distribution in the 79 combined nonexposed and 0 rad group cases was 73 (92.4%), 3 (3.8%), and 3 (3.8%) in categories I, II, and IV, respectively. Because of differing criteria for histological classification, this histological distribution is different from that described by Ueda *et al.* (*27*) for 95 cases of ovarian cancer in the Osaka district, of which 68 (71.6%), 7 (7.4%), and 19 (20.0%) were for categories I, II, and IV,

TABLE IV. Distribution of Ovarian Cancer by Histological Type and Exposure Dose

Histological type (WHO 1973)		Total		T65 dose in rad				
				0	1–99	100+	Unknown	NIC[a]
I.	Common epithelial tumors	121	(94.5%)	50	35	12	1	23
	A. Serous	61		26	17	7	1	10
	B. Mucinous	27		12	7	2	0	6
	C. Endometrioid	18		8	4	1	0	5
	D. Clear cell	9		2	3	2	0	2
	G. Undifferentiated carcinoma	2		0	2	0	0	0
	H. Unclassified malignancy	4		2	2	0	0	0
II.	Sex cord stromal tumors	4	(3.1%)	1	1	0	0	2
	A. Granulosa cell	4		1	1	0	0	2
IV.	Germ cell tumors	3	(2.3%)	0	0	0	0	3
	F. Teratomas	3		0	0	0	0	3
Total		128	(100.0%)	51	36	12	1	28

[a] Not in city ATB.

respectively (one case belonged to a category other than I–IV). These distributions should also be compared to that reported by Yaker and Benirschke (*29*) in 74 cases in the San Diego district, which was 66 (89.2%), 2 (2.7%), and 6 (8.1%), respectively.

The histological distribution of the 79 combined nonexposed and 0 rad group cases is not significantly different from that of the 49 cases exposed to 1 rad or more, namely, 48 carcinomas of category I and one granulosa cell tumor of category II. Of the 48 carcinomas among the exposed cases, serous adenocarcinoma accounted for 52.1%, followed in order by mucinous adenocarcinoma and endometrioid carcinoma. Of the 12 cases among those that were exposed to 100 or more rad, 7 were serous adenocarcinoma, 2 mucinous adenocarcinoma, 1 endometrioid carcinoma, and 2 clear cell carcinoma. Of 7 in the 12 cases exposed to 200 or more rad, 4 were serous adenocarcinoma, 1 mucinous adenocarcinoma, and 2 clear cell carcinoma. In 3 out of the 12 cases exposed to 300 or more rad, 2 were serous adenocarcinoma and 1 was clear cell carcinoma. Thus there is no evidence of different histological type of carcinoma with varying magnitude of exposure dose.

Consider next the issue of benign tumors of the ovary. It is plausible that the clinical recognition of such benign tumors may be somewhat related to the frequency of receiving professional medical care. Were this conjecture true, one might expect the frequency of recognized benign tumors to be higher in exposed individuals, especially in those exposed to large doses, as these individuals would likely have received more frequent and intense medical care than nonexposed persons (due to the A-bomb Survivors Medical Treatment Law, *etc.*). In the autopsied series, there would be no such bias in the recognition of benign tumors of the ovary. A study was thus undertaken on benign ovarian tumors from 106 autopsied LSS cases of which 89 cases (84.0%) were reviewed microscopically. As shown in Table V, the proportion of autopsied cases with benign ovarian tumors increases with increasing exposure dose, both with the group of all 106 ascertained benign tumor cases ($p<0.05$), and with the restricted subset of 89 microscopically reviewed cases, although statistical significance is not achieved in this latter group ($p>0.10$).

Because tumors were bilateral in 9 cases, the total number of tumors amount to 98 in the 89 histologically reviewed cases. The histological distribution of these 98 tumors

TABLE V. Age-adjusted Proportion of Subjects with Benign Ovarian Tumor Among Autopsied Subjects (per 1,000) by Exposure Dose

Method of ascertainment	Total	T65 dose in rad						Test[b]
		0	1–49	50–99	100+	Unknown	NIC[a]	
Total	34.8	26.3	38.8	47.6	58.8	30.6	27.8	
	(106)	(22)	(48)	(8)	(11)	(1)	(16)	$p<0.05$
Histologically	29.2	21.5	34.1	35.1	42.2	29.9	24.3	
reviewed cases	(89)	(18)	(42)	(6)	(8)	(1)	(14)	$p>0.10$

The number in parentheses is the number of subjects with benign ovarian tumor.
[a] Not in city ATB.
[b] Statistical test for linear increase with dose (excluding unknown and NIC).

TABLE VI. Distribution of Autopsied Benign Ovarian Tumors by Histological Type and Exposure Dose

Histological type (WHO 1973)	Total	T65 dose in rad				
		0	1–99	100+	Unknown	NIC[a]
I. Common epithelial tumors	60 (61.2%)	12	37	2	1	8
A. Serous	49	9	33	2	0	5
B. Mucinous	5	3	0	0	1	1
C. Endometrioid	1	0	1	0	0	0
E. Brenner	5	0	3	0	0	2
II. Sex cord stromal tumors	17 (17.3%)	3	8	3	0	3
b. Fibroma	16	2	8	3	0	3
c. Sclerosing stromal	1	1	0	0	0	0
IV. Germ cell tumors	21 (21.4%)	5	9	3	0	4
2. Mature cystic teratoma	19	3	9	3	0	4
3. Struma ovarii	2	2	0	0	0	0
Total	98 (100.0%)	20	54	8	1	15

[a] Not in city ATB.

is shown in Table VI. Of the 35 tumors occurring in the combined nonexposed and 0 rad groups, the number (and percentage) in categories I, II, and IV are 20 (57.1%), 6 (17.1%), and 9 (25.7%), respectively. This histologic distribution is not significantly different from that of the 63 tumors in cases exposed to 1 or more rad, namely, 40 (63.5%), 11 (17.5%), and 12 (19.0%) in categories I, II, IV, respectively. Comparison can also be made with other reported histologic distributions: 177 (45.2%), 20 (5.1%), and 193 (49.2%) among 392 tumors (including two cases in other than categories I–IV) in the Osaka district (*27*); 54 (46.6%), 14 (12.1%), and 48 (41.4%) among 116 tumors in San Diego (*29*); 637 (62.5%), 75 (7.4%), and 297 (29.1%) among 1,019 tumors (including 10 cases in other than categories I–IV) in Montreal (*2*). Thus, the distribution in this study does not differ significantly from reports mentioned above, except those in Osaka.

Experiments in radiation tumorigenesis have shown that ovarian tumors of several histological types can be induced in mice of various strains. For example, single dose whole-body irradiation of $(C57L \times A/He)F_1$ mice with gamma rays or neutrons induced various ovarian tumors, including luteoma, granulosa cell tumor, and adenoma (*28*). Similarly, single dose whole-body X-ray irradiation induced luteomas and adenomas in the ovaries of ddY/F and C3H/Tw mice (*12*).

It has been suggested that ionizing radiation primarily induces atrophy of follicles in the mouse ovary (*14*), and the consequent imbalanced hormonal environment, due to excessive gonadotropic hormone secretion, plays a significant role in the tumorigenesis of the ovary (*13*). In this regard, Furth (*8*) stated that a series of changes, namely, atrophy of the ovary due to radiation exposure, the secondary excess of gonadotrophic hormones, and changes in the response of cells that comprise the injured ovary, facilitate the development of ovarian tumors.

According to the study by Tokunaga *et al.* (*25*), breast cancer incidence in exposed females of Hiroshima and Nagasaki shows a linear dose response, and the age specific incidence of breast cancer exceeds that of breast cancer in the general female population. However, both the trend of the cumulative incidence with time and the histological distribution of breast cancer closely resemble that of breast cancer in general. These findings are consistent with the hypothesis that postexposure endogenous hormones act as tumor promoters in the genesis of breast cancer in A-bomb female survivors (*25*).

The pathological and epidemiological analyses described herein of the 194 cases of ovarian cancer that had occurred during 1950–80 among LSS members strongly suggest that the incidence of ovarian cancer was enhanced by A-bomb exposure; moreover, the radiation-related excess of ovarian cancer appears to be highest in women less than 20 years of age when exposed, with these women having the longest latent period compared to the older age groups. The histological distribution of cancer types among exposed individuals appears not very different from that seen in the general population. As for benign ovarian neoplasms, the analysis of 106 autopsy subjects depicts a trend of increasing radiation-related tumor excess with increasing dose among the exposed cases, though the trend is not statistically significant when observation was limited to the histologically reviewed cases.

From experimental findings concerning the induction of ovarian tumors by ionizing radiation and from recent analysis of breast carcinogenesis in exposed females of Hiroshima and Nagasaki, one might deduce that radiation injury in association with secondary excess of gonadotrophic hormones is an important causative factor in the development of ovarian tumors in the Hiroshima and Nagasaki female survivors; the pathological and epidemiological findings detailed herein are consistent with this hypothesis. Further follow-up studies should therefore be made on females who were exposed to the A-bomb at the younger ages, particularly at ages less than 20 years when exposed.

REFERENCES

1. Anderson, M. R. and Jackson, S. H. Long term follow-up of patients with menorrhagia treated by irradiation. *Br. J. Radiol.*, **44**, 295–298 (1971).
2. Beck, R. P. and Latour, J.P.A. Review of 1019 benign ovarian neoplasms. *Obstet. Gynecol.*, **16**, 479–482 (1960).
3. Boice, J. D., Jr., Day, N. E., Andersen, A., Brinton, L. A., Brown, P., Choi, N. W., Clarke, E. A., Colemen, M. P., Curtis, R. E., Flannery, J. T., Hakama, M., Hakulinen, T., Howe, G. R., Jensen, O. M., Kleinerman, R. A., Magnin, D., Magnus, K., Makela, K., Malker, B., Miller, A. B., Nelson, N., Patterson, C. C., Pettersson, F., Pompe-Kirn, V., Primic-Zakelc, M., Prior, P., Ravnihar, P., Skeet, R. G., Skjerven, J. E., Smith, P. G., Sok, N., Spengler, R. F., Storm, H. H., Tomkins, G.W.O., Wall, C., and Weinstock, R. Cancer risk following radiotherapy of cervical cancer. *In* "Radiation Carcinogenesis: Epidemiology and Biological Significance: Progress in Cancer Research, Vol 26.," ed.

SUBJECT INDEX